YOGA FOR WOMEN

YOGA FOR WOMEN
A Gentler Strength

Paddy O'Brien has practised and taught yoga for many years and also runs a personnel training consultancy. She runs general yoga classes and ante- and post-natal yoga classes. She has written many magazine articles and is the author of several books including *Birth and our Bodies* and *Your Life After Birth*. She lives in Berkshire with her partner and five children.

YOGA FOR WOMEN

A GENTLER STRENGTH

Paddy O'Brien

Illustrations by Su Eaton
Photographs by Hanya Chlala

Thorsons
An Imprint of HarperCollins*Publishers*

Thorsons
An Imprint of HarperCollins*Publishers*
77–85 Fulham Palace Road,
Hammersmith, London W6 8JB
1160 Battery Street,
San Francisco, California 94111–1213

First published by Thorsons 1991 as 'A Gentler Strength'
This edition published 1994
3 5 7 9 10 8 6 4

© 1991 and 1994 Paddy O'Brien

Paddy O'Brien asserts the moral right
to be identified as the author of this work

A catalogue record for this book
is available from the British Library

ISBN 1 85538 426 4

Typeset by Harper Phototypesetters Limited,
Northampton, England
Printed in Great Britain by
Scotprint Ltd, Musselburgh

CONTENTS

Dedication   vii
Acknowledgements   ix
Introduction   xi

1 BACKGROUND TO YOGA   1
Clothes and Equipment   1
How Much to Do, When to Do It   2
Choosing a Class   2
What are the Origins of Yoga?   3
The Benefits   4
How to Use This Book   5

2 PRACTICE GUIDELINES AND BASIC POSES   6
Practice Guidelines   6
Programme Design   6
Basic Session   7
    Standing Poses   8
    Back Bends   19
    Sitting Poses   22
    Awareness of Breathing   29
    Meditation   31
    Yantra and Mandala   33

3 LIFE PASSAGES   36
Adolescence   37
Menstrual Cycle   41
Pregnancy   46
The Post-natal Months   51
The Menopause   55

4 LIFE EVENTS   59
   Alone or Separated   59
   In a Loving Partnership   62
   Overstressed   65
   Understressed   69
   Feeling Fragile   70
   Very Fit   71

5 IMAGE AND LIFESTYLE   75
   Eating, Size and Weight   75
   Chakra, Colour and Sound   78
   Yama and Niyama – On Not Going to Extremes   82
   Yoga Nidra   86
   Visualization   87

   Conclusion   91
   Further Reading   93
   Index   95

DEDICATION

TO S.J. O'B WITH MY LOVE

ACKNOWLEDGEMENTS

My thanks are due to all the yoga teachers whose classes I have attended over the years, but especially recently to Barbara Griggs and Arjan Shahani, both of whom work constantly for understanding and exploration in yoga. I'd also like to thank all the women who have attended my classes and shared their experiences and reflections so fully.

Finally, my thanks and love to Tim.

INTRODUCTION

This book is intended as a source and introduction to yoga for women young and old, fit and unfit, beginners and experienced practitioners alike. Yoga is a huge field of deep and subtle experience and study: here I have tried simply to reflect on the aspects of yoga which feel to me to be particularly important for women.

We inhabit our beautiful women's bodies in a sexist culture in a polluted and violent world, and are often exiled both from a sense of our own beauty, and from a clear view of how to live with the dangers around us.

The pressures placed on women by our society force us to become strong in any case, but that strength is often one full of stress and tension. In the practice of yoga there is a chance to find a gentler strength with which to flow with our lives.

I first came across yoga 20 years ago completely by chance. It was the kind of chance that makes you wonder why you worry about making major decisions, because the choices which have the most radical long-term effects so often happen apparently at random: yoga changed and is still changing my life.

The impact of a teenage pregnancy had left me heavy and unfit in body and chaotic in spirit, and I had never been adept in any way at dance, gymnastics or games. However, my yoga teacher constantly emphasized the non-competitive aspect of yoga, making clear that the important part was simply to be fully present in your body, mind and spirit, at the time.

Very, very slowly, I became more supple, stronger, and lighter. At times I felt peaceful too.

Yoga has not made my life simple, or made my body a constant or ideal size and shape, or made my heart always calm. It has, however, always been with me, always been available, always been a companionable source of strength and ideas. I have done yoga in a bleak way during bleak parts of my life, and in an idyllic and joyful way when that has been the flavour of my existence.

Yoga practice has enriched my life however full or empty of grace I felt at the time I did it.

That is how it has been for me. Since everyone's experience is different I cannot tell how it will be for you. You may undergo great changes and upheavals, or startling revelations, or slow and quiet growth, or such phases may alternate. You may find in yourself qualities you never knew you had, your body may change in size or demeanour, or perhaps nothing at all will happen for some time. You do not know until you try.

I hope the ideas and suggestions in this book make a good starting place for you if you have not thought of yoga before. If you are already a student of yoga, I hope you will find material here that will interact in a new and positive way with your current thinking and practice.

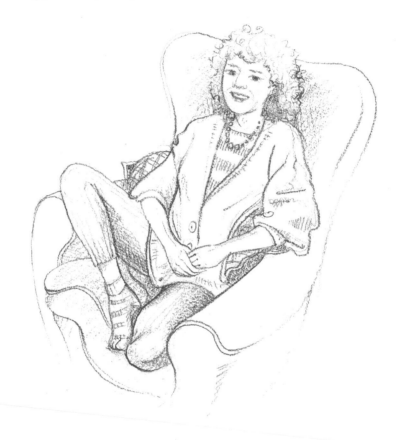

CHAPTER ONE

BACKGROUND TO YOGA

The word 'yoga' comes from a Sanskrit word which means 'yoke' or 'something which joins or connects'. Some of the practices of yoga are known as 'hatha yoga'. 'Ha' is the sun and 'tha' is the moon, so 'hatha yoga' is 'what joins the sun and the moon'. In other words, yoga is a way of joining together and reintegrating opposites, contradictions, fragmented and broken parts of life, the yin and the yang, the warm and the cold, the swift and the slow, the sun and the moon.

Most women will recognize immediately how they have to fulfil many contradictory roles and reconcile many opposites in their lives, and see, therefore, that yoga is a wonderful resource for women. It works on many levels and you can enter into it in a cheerful open-hearted way at whatever level you feel is appropriate for you. As it becomes part of your life it will bring a deep respect and love for your own, and therefore everybody else's, body and indeed for the whole physical world, although you do not have to be uncomfortably solemn. Of course there are serious moments in the practice of yoga, but there is plenty of humour and pleasure too, so start in a light and hopeful frame of mind.

CLOTHES AND EQUIPMENT

You don't need any special equipment to begin with – all that is necessary is a clean, comfortable space and a clean blanket.

In warm weather it is pleasant to practise outside. Take care of your balance outside – indoors one unconsciously refers to the verticals and horizontals of a room in order to balance; outdoors you may feel strangely wobbly at first.

You do not need any special clothes either. You should work in bare feet both because you are less likely to slip, and so that you can really feel all of your footprint on the floor. Your feet will gradually become sensitive, flexible and expressive, and you will feel the full meaning and security of the phrase 'having your feet on the ground'. Wear something which is not tight around the waist and which allows you a full range of movement and stretch in both arms and legs. If you enjoy your yoga you may want to buy a leotard or track suit or some soft trousers and tops for your practice. Instinct will guide you to choose colours which are expressive of you. In cool weather keep your practice space warm and wear plenty of layers so that you can take off layers and put them on again as you need to. Do not be misled into thinking that because you are not sweating and breathless you are not warming up and cooling down when you do your yoga: wrap up and keep warm so that your muscles can cool down slowly and gradually.

HOW MUCH TO DO, WHEN TO DO IT

Some people find it useful to practise at the same time daily or on whichever days thay choose as their 'yoga days', as they feel it keeps a steady rhythm of practice going. New students worry a great deal about how much practice to do and how they are going to 'motivate' themselves to 'keep it up', but this really is not a problem. The impulse which interests you in the first place, which prompts you to work from books and go to class, will keep you going for the first few months of your involvement with yoga. This early period is when it feels like something separate that you do a little self-consciously – 'Now I am going to do my yoga exercises'. Later on it will be the most natural thing in the world to go and do it, and you will not have to 'motivate' yourself any more than you have to motivate yourself to eat or breathe. As a rule of thumb for how long to spend on your personal practise at home, think about what is practicable within the shape of your life as it is at the moment. Anything between half an hour and two hours for a session, and anything between once and six times a week, would be sensible parameters. (Have at least one 'rest day' a week.) If you go to class and 'can't motivate yourself' to practise at home, then don't practise at home for the moment, as you obviously aren't ready to, for whatever reason. Students make tremendous progress, even when one *knows* they are not doing postures at all from one class to the next. Practising yoga *does* change you, and the

impulse to *not* practise may sometimes be a hesitation in facing up to some of the changes, or a desire to slow down the rate of change. That is all right. When the time is right you will do more. This attitude of finding out from inside how much to do, rather than having it imposed from the outside, is new to most of us who have grown up in the West. However, far from leading to the floppiness and passivity which might at first seem likely, it actually generates a self-reliance and toughness. It is very important for us as women, who may well have been taught and conditioned since our time as little girls, to look for approval and validation from others. Yoga gives the responsibility to *you* to decide how long is long enough to work, how hard is hard enough to try, how well is well done. Of course one makes mistakes, sometimes painfully, but the inner strength and self-respect that come with this discipline of deciding for yourself what is your honest best on any particular day can be a wonderful antidote to a lifetime of waiting for praise or blame from parents, teachers, bosses, partners, or other powerful figures in one's life.

CHOOSING A CLASS

'When the student is ready, the teacher will appear.' There is often a striking serendipity in the ways in which people 'run into' exactly the right teacher for themselves. These ways can range from sitting next to them on the bus and, contrary to the habit of a lifetime, starting to chat to them, to walking a different way home from usual and seeing a class through a window and feeling 'drawn in'; there are all sorts of other apparent coincidences which bring together the student and the teacher who are right for one another. However, some of us have to find our teachers through the more prosaic means of contacting dance and exercise studios or yoga and fitness centres and making enquiries! When you find a class that seems to be at the right time, the right place, and the right level for you, see if you can go to just a few sessions first of all to see how you get on. Talk to the teacher about his or her background. Yoga teachers are used to being asked who their teachers were and are, what styles they have been influenced by and what their qualifications are. Mention anything special about your body, particularly any current or past back injuries or whiplash neck injuries, raised blood pressure, detached retina, or if you are pregnant. None of these conditions will prevent you from doing yoga, but there are some postures you should omit or modify, so your teacher needs to know.

The atmosphere of the class should be calm and cheerful, and there should be no sense whatever of competition or display. The teacher should be calm, competent and respectful of the students. She or he should be moving around the class at least some of the time and helping students individually – not just demonstrating at the front all the time. Apart from those guidelines, you are going to have to follow your own intuition about whether you are in the class which is right for you. There is considerable variation from class to class in the emphasis and attitude of the teacher and the style of posture practised. We all write in the same alphabet but we all have unique handwriting. The yoga postures may be the same, but everyone has a slightly different way of doing and interpreting them. You must decide for yourself whether any particular class rings true for you.

With those points in mind, do go to class as well as working from the book if you can. Your teacher can see you in all three dimensions and from the back, which you cannot! She can therefore help you make adjustments which you would be unlikely to discover yourself. It is fun to work with other students and to learn from each other as well as sharing the ups and downs, the hilarities and frustrations which will certainly be part of the experience.

WHAT ARE THE ORIGINS OF YOGA?

Yoga is an ancient practice which originated in India. One of the oldest known pictures of someone practising a yoga pose is carved on a stone seal dating from about 2500 BC, and was found on the site of Mohenjo-Daro in the Indus Valley. Yoga was first mentioned as a techique in a collection of hymns and philosophical poetry called the *Vedas*, which were written cumulatively over a period of 2,000 years and transmitted first orally and then in a written form. In the sixth century BC the *Bhagavadgita* was written. It is one part of a long epic poem called the *Mahabharata* and describes a dialogue between the god Krishna and the warrior Arjuna about the philosophy and practice of yoga, and it also discusses methods by which the yoga way of life can be lived.

In the second century AD, the *Yoga Sutras of Patanjali* were collected and written down. *Sutra* means 'thread' (the same root word as 'suture') – the short aphorisms of the *Sutras* must be unravelled like thread to be understood, and woven together to make a whole, like threads woven into a patterned fabric, in order to make a full picture. *Patanjali* describes yoga as an eight-fold path. The eight paths are:

1 Laws of Life – *Yama*
2 Rules for Living – *Niyama*

3 Postures – *Asana*
4 Breathing Exercises – *Pranayama*
5 Withdrawing the Senses – *Pratayahara*
6 Concentration – *Dharana*
7 Meditation – *Dhyana*
8 Peace of Mind – *Samadhi*

These are discussed more fully in Chapters 5 and 6.

The huge time scale of the development of yoga is helpful when first coming to yoga in later years, or when one has neglected yoga for some time and is feeling stale or guilty. Yoga has been around for thousands of years. It will wait another couple of months or years for you if you need it to. It's not going to vanish overnight.

Many different styles of yoga are practised in the twentieth century. You will probably find yourself temperamentally, aesthetically, or spiritually drawn to one or other style.
A teacher who has trained in the *Iyengar* style will look very different in the postures and will work in a very different way from one who is strongly influenced by the *Desikachar* approach or the *Sivananda* group's methods.

Claims and counter-claims about which is the 'best' way are not appropriate. So long as your teacher is safe, accurate and, as far as you can tell, has an authentic attitude and personal integrity, you must study the method with which you feel most 'at one'.

THE BENEFITS

Anybody who is interested in health, fitness and exercise will have spent the 1980s reading book after book about this or that system which makes stupendous claims for the method described. After exposure to all this, most of us have developed a defensive layer of cynicism. 'Oh yeah,' we think. 'Funny how *all* these techniques are supposed to be the best, the quickest, make you lose the most weight, gain the most confidence, and transform yourself the most radically.' Even more embarrassing than straight hype is hype plus obvious sniping at rival fitness programmes. In this context, how are we to describe the benefits of yoga?

Briefly, the physical benefits of yoga practice are:

• enhanced flexibility of muscles and joints
• enhanced muscular strength and power
• improved heart and lung function
• toning of immune system, glands, such as the pituitary and thyroid, and of the digestive systems

The emotional benefits are:

• an ability to rebalance stresses
• an ability to get in touch with inner peace

In a way, that's all. What more could one want! There are other aspects, though, which make yoga particularly worthwhile and attractive for women. You can do yoga in all sorts of periods of your life. You can do it while you are fragile, vulnerable, undermined or exhausted, as well as when you are confident, exuberant and celebrating your strength. You don't have to be fit or supple to start with. You start from where you are at this moment.

Yoga is not a competitive form of exercise. There is terrible cultural pressure on women to be competitive in all sorts of areas, particularly weight, size and appearance. It is a great relief and pleasure to find a style of exercise that is loving and cooperative, that tunes into and enhances your own rhythms rather than imposing artificial stresses and rhythms upon you. It is a real way out of the 'rat race' of competitive living.

Although many of us begin yoga as a fitness programme, it is more than that. There is little need to say much about the compassion, peace and inspiration yoga brings. It does it anyway, whether you speak or think consciously about it or not. By concentrating clearly, steadily and with love on your own body, insights and changes arise, sometimes obvious and spectacular, more often perhaps, subtle and diffuse. When you are making a beginning with yoga, you need not bother overmuch about these ideas. In a few months or years you will begin to look back and see what they mean to you.

If you are a long-time practitioner you will know about these positive experiences. You probably also know the long deserts and darknesses, the plateaux where nothing happens, where your body won't open or strengthen any more and your spirit sags and drifts without inspiration. We all experience those times, too. Although they make no sense at the time perhaps they are the emptiness that balance the fullness, the darkness that balances the light. Most people who have practised for a long time have had such internal struggles and despair. They may be unable to practise and unable to work out why or to talk about why for weeks or months, but they will come out of it eventually. This experience of episodes of

blankness is common to all disciplines where the body is used expressively and exploratively, such as dance and the martial arts, as well as yoga. It must be in some way necessary, and it passes in time.

HOW TO USE THIS BOOK

The second chapter of this book explains and illustrates a basic series of yoga postures, which you could use as a core for your practice. The following chapters look at particular physical events and processes, and particular life events we may pass through as women, and suggest postures which may be useful at those times.

However, use the book creatively and intuitively once you have begun to feel at home with yoga. Within the guidelines of safety and balance (discussed fully in Chapter 2), you should design and evolve your own programmes.

The final chapters discuss more fully the philosophical background of yoga for women who want to reflect on and read more deeply into those aspects.

While this book is pleasant to browse through and look at, let it lead you into action too. As Swami Sivananda has said, 'an ounce of practice is worth a ton of theory': as soon as you feel you've absorbed enough to do so, begin to do some yoga for yourself, and enjoy the journey of exploration.

CHAPTER TWO

PRACTICE GUIDELINES
AND BASIC POSES

Here is a basic sequence of yoga poses or 'asanas' which you can use as a basis for designing your own practice.

The word 'asana' means 'seat' – and this means that it should be a comfortable position. When you first try out some of these postures you may find it amazing to think they could ever be positions of ease; however, in time, all these positions become pleasant and comfortable and the stretching sensation becomes as pleasant as an exhilarating waking-up stretch on a beautiful morning.

This sequence will take about 45 minutes at first as you will only spend a short time in each stretch. As time goes on you will find you settle for longer in each position, and this will expand the practice time to something between an hour and a quarter and an hour and a half. Even if you only have 10 or 15 minutes to spend on yoga, concentrate fully, move carefully and well, slip into your yoga frame of mind, and you will emerge refreshed as if you have had a cleansing shower after being grubby or a drink of water after feeling very thirsty.

PRACTICE GUIDELINES

- Move into each position slowly and carefully.
- Pay attention to what is going on in your body.
- Go to your own comfortable maximum – feel a stretch, but not a strain.
- Exhale as you stretch into a pose.
- Do not compete with anyone, *even yourself.*

Experience the posture fully, observe what you are feeling in it. It is through this attentive 'listening' to your body that development comes.

PROGRAMME DESIGN

To choose a balanced sequence of asanas you need a:

- 'Centred' pose (e.g. *tadasana* or *vrksasana*).
- Side stretch (e.g. *trikonasana* or *parsvakonasana*).
- Forward bend (e.g. *prasrita padottanasana* or *paschimottanasana*).
- Back bend (e.g. *bhujangasana* or *ustrasana*).
- Upside-down pose – except during menstrual periods (e.g. *sarvangasana* or *sirsasana* and variations).
- Relaxation (*savasana*).

Never miss *savasana*. If you have only 15 minutes to spend on yoga, spend 3 or 4 on relaxation. Dynamic stretching poses give us an outward strength, but only *savasana* can put you in touch with your inner strength and resources.

BASIC SESSION

Here is a basic programme which provides a balanced cross-section of asanas.

CENTRING

- Sit cross-legged on the floor.
- Sit on the centre of your pelvic floor, *not* back on your tailbone.
- Check with a hand on your abdomen. When correctly positioned, your abdomen is long. When incorrectly positioned your abdomen is squashed.
- Lift your spine and the crown of your head.

- Open your chest and release your shoulders.
- Breathe slowly and deeply.
- As you breathe, think 'breathe away tension, breathe in peace'.

The reason for sitting quietly at the beginning of your session is to ensure that you have gathered together your awareness and concentration and cleared your mind of irrelevant thoughts and mood-swings before you begin. If you remember to do this you will make fewer mistakes and very much reduce your chances of injury from jerking out of posture or making an awkward or incoherent movement because part of your mind is elsewhere. You will also have a much more satisfying time with your yoga if you are fully present with it.

When your mind is clear and settled and your body is poised, you will feel ready to 'come to' and move into the postures. Allow yourself to become aware of the place you are in, of

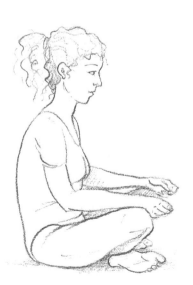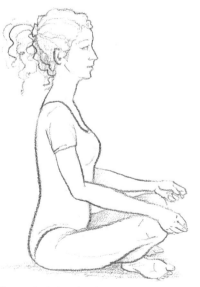

Difference between sitting centrally and sitting back on tail bone

the things around you. Let your breathing come back to an everyday level. Rub your hands together to warm them, then cover your face with your warmed hands and separate your fingers. Blink your eyes open behind your hands and let them get used to the light, before floating your hands down into your lap.

VARIATIONS

If your knees feel too stiff at first to relax in this position, try sitting with one or two cushions under each knee. If there is a stiffness in your hips, try a firm cushion, or your blanket folded up under your hips so that the back of your bottom is lifted an inch or two off the ground. If you are still too uncomfortable to sit and be calm and still your thoughts with these variations, then stretch your legs out in front of you, hip distance apart, and gently bent. Try the cross-legged position again, with cushions if necessary, in a few weeks' time. In a few weeks or months it will eventually become accessible to you.

Standing Poses

TADASANA – MOUNTAIN POSE

- Wriggle your toes, rise up on tiptoe a few times, then bring your feet together.
- Feel your legs straighten and strengthen.
- Tuck your tailbone under and lift your abdomen lightly.
- Open your chest and relax your shoulders.
- Lengthen through your spine and up through the crown of your head.
- Keep your face soft, and breathe slowly and steadily.

This is a lovely pose which grows in meaning the more you practise it. Beginning as a way of standing well, it becomes a pose in which you can sense your connection with the earth, your strength, your balance and resilience.

In this and all your yoga poses, lift your abdomen lightly. As women, we often have a very emotional relationship with our abdomens. Fashion dictates that we should have tight, boyish tummies. We dedicate ourselves to sit-ups, crunches, leg-raising, anything to eliminate any womanly roundness or softness. It is genuinely difficult to disentangle the positive desire to have strong healthy abdominal muscles and to dispense with layers of fat that feel sluggish and unpleasant, from a much more anxious desire to re-create our bodies in the image of the advertising industry's fantasy woman.

Yoga will certainly strengthen your abdomen and tighten it if it has a lot of accumulated fat which is not doing anything positive for you. However, this change is not arrived at by hating your body, but by keeping it light and active.

BENEFITS

- Improved balance.
- A sense of strength.
- Awareness of your physicality.

When you feel it is time to move out of *tadasana*, step your feet apart a little way and relax – but don't collapse.

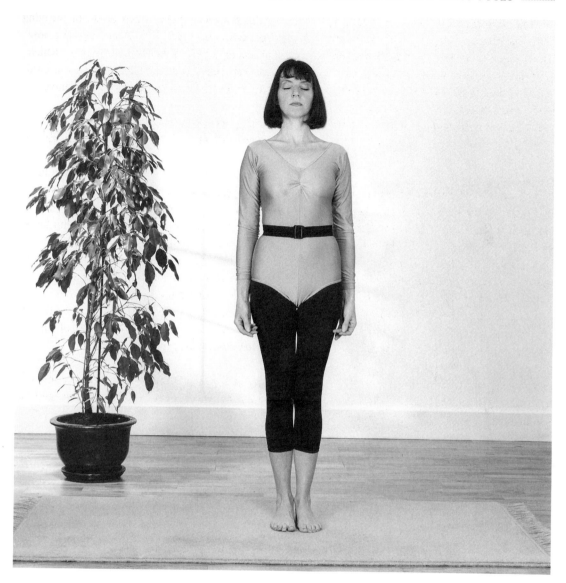

Tadasana (mountain pose)

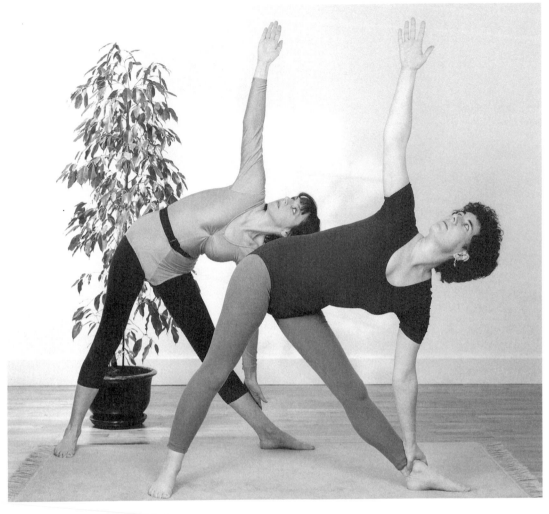

Trikonasana (triangle pose)

TRIKONASANA – TRIANGLE POSE

- Step your feet 3–3½ feet apart.
- Turn your left foot in, right foot out, right heel in line with left instep.
- Hips face the front.
- Inhale, raise your arms out to the sides at shoulder level.
- Exhale, relax your shoulders and stretch along your arms out to your finger tips.
- Inhale again, and as you exhale, stretch out to the right, and down to the right place for you today. Place your hand on knee, ankle or the floor, whichever is appropriate.
- Turn and look at the upper thumb with the lower eye.

BENEFITS

- Extending limbs and spine.
- Sensing the balance between hips and shoulders.
- Strengthening legs and abdomen.
- Freshening and toning the face.

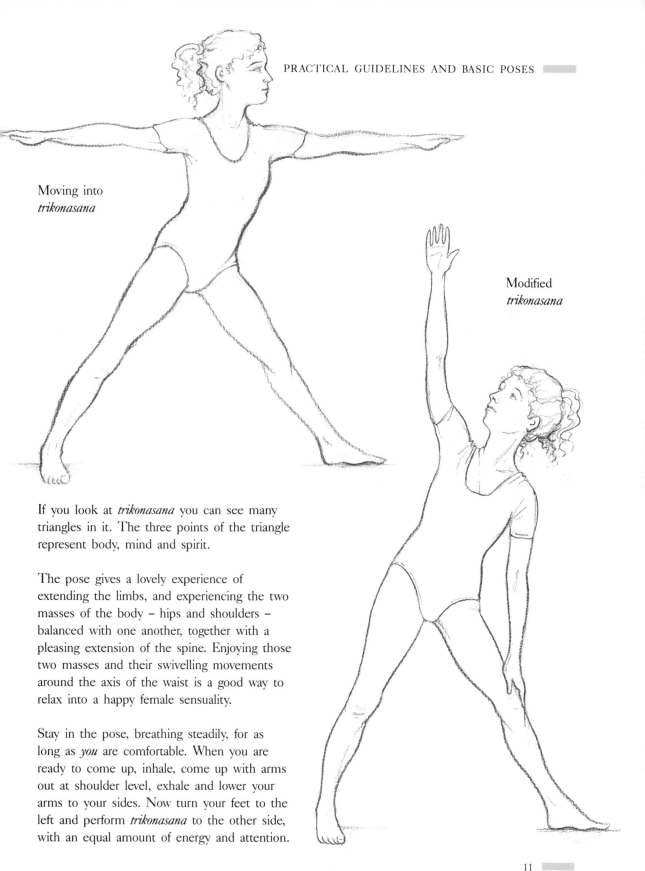

Moving into
trikonasana

Modified
trikonasana

If you look at *trikonasana* you can see many triangles in it. The three points of the triangle represent body, mind and spirit.

The pose gives a lovely experience of extending the limbs, and experiencing the two masses of the body – hips and shoulders – balanced with one another, together with a pleasing extension of the spine. Enjoying those two masses and their swivelling movements around the axis of the waist is a good way to relax into a happy female sensuality.

Stay in the pose, breathing steadily, for as long as *you* are comfortable. When you are ready to come up, inhale, come up with arms out at shoulder level, exhale and lower your arms to your sides. Now turn your feet to the left and perform *trikonasana* to the other side, with an equal amount of energy and attention.

PARSVAKONASANA – SIDE FLANK STRETCH

Parsva means side, and *kona* means angle.

- Step your feet 4–4½ feet apart. Turn your left foot in, right foot out, right heel in line with left instep.
- Inhale, raise your arms out to the sides at shoulder level.
- Exhale, bend your right knee, forming a right angle between thigh and calf. Do not shoot the right knee out beyond the foot. Keep the calf vertical.
- Inhale again and as you exhale, stretch out to the right. Either rest your elbow on your right knee, or take your hand to the floor behind your right foot. Take your left arm up over your head to form a continuous line from your outer left foot to your left fingertips.
- Turn and look up from under your upper arm.
- Make sure your hips face the front. Keep your face and throat relaxed and breathe steadily.

BENEFITS

- Strengthening the legs.
- Flexibility in the waist.
- Loosening the shoulders.
- Freeing up the chest.
- Vitality to the whole body.

Stay in the pose, breathing steadily for as long as *you* are comfortable. When you are ready to come up, inhale, come up with arms out at shoulder level, exhale, and lower your arms to your sides. Then turn your feet the other way and practise with equal energy and attention on the other side.

Preparation for *parsvakonasana*

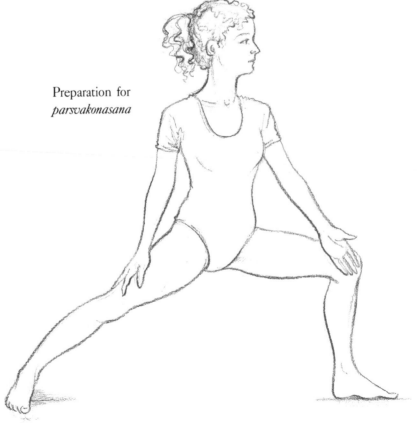

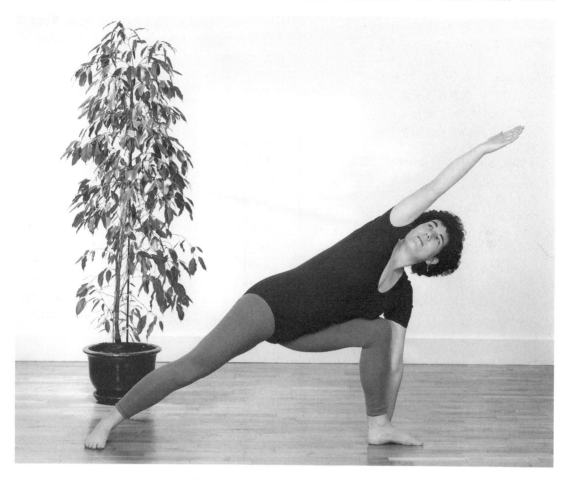

Parsvakonasana (side flank stretch)

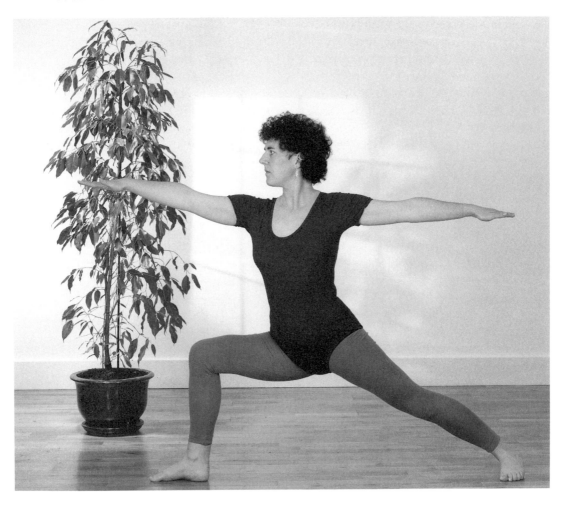

Virabhadrasana (warrior pose II)

VIRABHADRASANA – WARRIOR POSE II

- Step your feet 4–4½ feet apart. Turn your left foot in, right foot out, right heel in line with left instep.
- Make sure your hips and chest face squarely to the front.
- Inhale, and raise your arms out to the sides at shoulder level. Exhale, relax your shoulders, and stretch out to your fingertips.
- Inhale again, and as you exhale, bend your right knee, forming a right angle between thigh and calf. Do not shoot the right knee out over the foot.
- Turn and look at your right fingertips.
- Check that your arms are parallel to the ground, not inclining either up or down.
- Breathe steadily and keep your face and throat relaxed.

BENEFITS

- Strengthens legs and arms.
- A feeling of expansion in chest and hips.
- Enhanced balance.
- A sense of power and confidence.

Only stay in the pose as long as is right for you. When you are ready, inhale and straighten your legs, exhale, turn to the front and lower your arms. *Virabhadra* was a fierce and courageous warrior. As you move into the posture imagine yourself poised on your horse like *Virabhadra*, ready to ride into battle. Take pride as a woman in the many, many battles you have fought, both for yourself, and on behalf of other people.

VRKSASASANA – TREE POSE

If you feel insecure when you start this pose, use a chair or the wall for support.

- Stand in *tadasana*.
- Bend your left knee, and keeping your hips open and your knee well back, place your left foot on the side of either your right

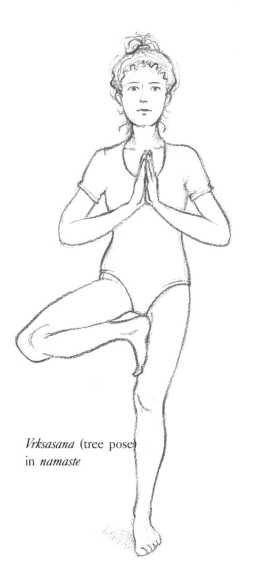

Vrksasana (tree pose) in *namaste*

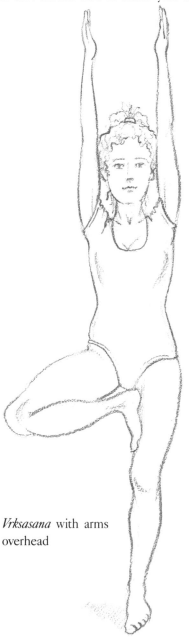

Vrksasana with arms overhead

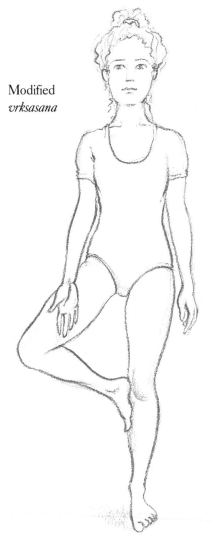

Modified
vrksasana

BENEFITS

- Improved poise and balance.
- A sense of steadiness and calm.
- Increased flexibility in the hips.

When you have spent enough time for you on one foot, exhale, lower your arms and release your foot. Hug towards you the leg you stood on, to release any tension in the thigh. Now practise, with equal attention and focus, balancing on the other leg.

PRASARITA PADOTTANASANA – WIDE STRIDE STRETCH

- Step your feet 4–4½ feet apart, feet parallel, with toes pointing forwards. Feel your feet are in good contact with the ground.
- Place your hands on your hips, inhale and stand tall.
- Exhale and stretch forwards, hinging at the hip, not the waist, keeping your back flat. When you cannot stretch forwards any more, start to stretch down.
- At your comfortable maximum, release the back of your neck and let your head be heavy, rest your hands or elbows, hands and head on the floor, or if you cannot reach yet, hold on to opposite elbows and simply hang.
- Keep a firm footing and keep the back and the front of your body long and free.

When you want to come out of the posture, wriggle your feet in a few inches. Breathing in, lift your head and exhaling, press your abdomen back towards your spine, and come up.

ankle, your right knee or tucked right in to the top of the right thigh, whichever is possible for you.

- Focus your gaze on a specific point in front of you. This will help you to balance.
- Either place your hands palm to palm in front of your heart, or stretch your arms up vertically, palms facing in.
- Draw strength up from under the ground into your feet, your legs, your torso, head and arms, right up to your fingertips.
- Breathe steadily with your face and throat relaxed.

VARIATION
If you have a lower back injury do not stretch all the way down in this pose. Simply go

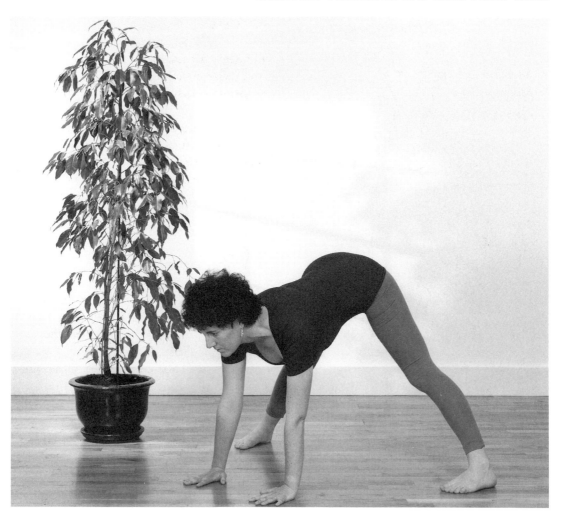

Prasarita padottanasana (wide stride stretch)

Advanced *prasarita*
padottanasana

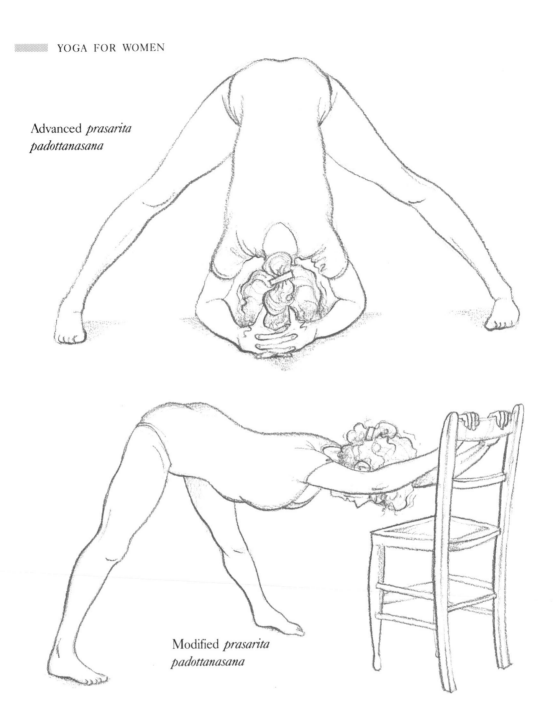

Modified *prasarita*
padottanasana

forwards until your torso is parallel to the
floor, and rest your hands with arms extended,
or folded arms, on a heavy piece of furniture
(a work top or heavy table which will not
slip). Concentrate on spreading your back
broad and flat, and strengthening your

abdominal muscles by flexing them back
towards your spine. Feel your legs strong,
stretched and lifting. When you want to come
out of your stretch, inhale and lift your head,
then exhaling, *walk towards the support* so you
do not stress your back when coming up.

Back Bends

These two back bends open and stretch the front of your body, and also flex the spine in a backwards stretch. Be careful and observant of your body in these postures and do not go any faster than your body wants to go. Do not get discouraged if you feel stiff and immobile, as little by little the impossible happens, and where you started off feeling like a block of concrete, you will eventually feel light, springy and flexible.

You should read carefully the following advice before starting practise on any back bends.

- Do not do powerful back bending postures in the second and third trimesters of pregnancy unless you are already very experienced in yoga.
- If you have recently experienced back strain or injury, move very slowly and attentively into a gentler version of any back bending posture, and avoid holding your breath.
- Be sure to do the counter posture, praying stretch (pages 48–9) and release your back fully.
- An astounding 80 per cent of adults in the affluent West have back problems of one kind or another. Careful practise of forward and back bends (it is important to do both) is protective of the health of your spine.

BHUJANGASANA – COBRA POSE

Bhujanga is a serpent. *Bhujangasana* is often called the cobra pose, as the upper body eventually lifts off the ground like a cobra preparing to strike.

- Lie face downwards on the floor with your knees and feet together.
- Place your palms on the floor on either side of your chest with your fingers pointing forwards.
- Lengthen the back of your neck and put your face to the floor. Inhale.
- As you exhale, lift your face from the floor, and then lift chest and belly off the floor if you can.
- Keep your shoulders relaxed. Only come up as far as is right for you for today.
- Breathe steadily as long as is comfortable (only a few seconds at first). Keep your face and throat relaxed.
- When you have had enough, exhale and flow forwards and down onto the ground.

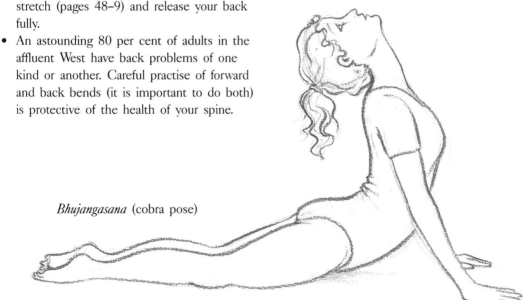

Bhujangasana (cobra pose)

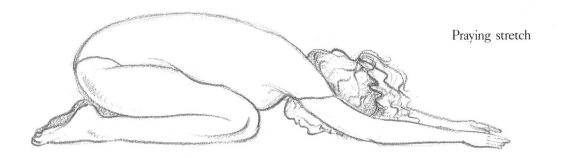

Praying stretch

- Turn your head to one side and rest until your heartbeat and breathing have returned to normal.

Repeat *bhujangasana* one more time, then

- Push up onto all fours.
- Separate your knees and bring your toes together.
- Exhale and sit back as far as you can towards your heels and inch your fingertips further forwards.
- Keep the back *and* the front of your body as long and free as you can.
- Breathe steadily in this stretch (praying stretch). Use it to take any stress out of your back after all your back bends.

VARIATION

If you are too stiff at first to fold forwards along your thighs, sit back on your heels, and fold your arms onto the seat of a chair, resting your head down onto your arms and gradually increasing the flexibility in your spine.

USTRASANA – CAMEL POSE

This is a more intense back bend.

- Kneel on the floor, knees together and insteps on the ground.
- Inhale, stretch upwards, and lengthen out your hips till your thighs are vertical.
- Exhale, lean your upper body backwards and reach back to hold onto your heels.
- Keep your thighs vertical and think of holding your torso parallel to the floor.
- Let your head fall back, and think of keeping your neck long.
- Remain there for a few seconds breathing steadily, keeping your face and throat soft.
- When you are ready to come up, think *abdomen* strength, not back strength.
- Inhale and come up, exhale and go straight down into praying stretch.

VARIATION

At first you may find the pose easier with your knees a few inches apart and your toes curled under and pressing into the floor.

These back bends are stimulating for your spine, and also make the front of your body feel fresh and alive. Another quality of back bending postures is that they help to recover movements and positions which we all enjoyed as children.

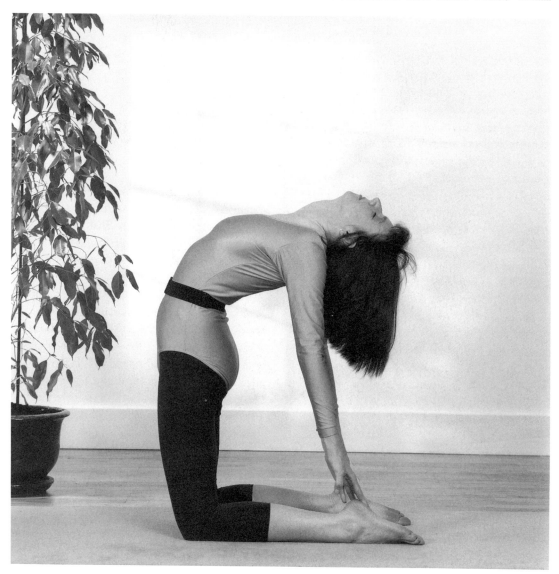

Ustrasana (camel pose)

Sitting Poses

Sitting poses bring a lightness and flexibility to the hips and legs, and many of them give a composed and comfortable position for the body to rest in while you practise meditation or *pranayama*. Many of them can simply become ordinary ways of sitting when you sit on the floor: and sitting on the floor more frequently will increase your flexibility and mobility anyhow.

DANDASANA – STAFF POSE

- Sit on the floor with your legs extended straight in front of you, heels pushing away.
- Pull your hips back to make sure you are sitting on the centre of your pelvic floor.
- Lift up through the whole spine, lift the crown of your head and keep your chin in so that the back of your neck is long.
- Lift your abdomen and relax your shoulders.

- Place the palms of your hands on the floor at hip level, fingers pointing forwards.
- Either close your eyes and focus within, or take your gaze to the floor beyond your feet.
- Breathe steadily, keeping your face and throat relaxed. Stay in this pose for anything up to a couple of minutes, then exhale and relax but do not collapse.

Dandasana inculcates in the body a habit of sitting tall with the spine stretched up and the abdomen lifting and free, so that the circulation and the workings of the soft inner organs are improved.

VARIATION

If *dandasana* is so uncomfortable that it is impossible to hold it at all – and this does sometimes happen at first – fold your blanket into a firm rectangular block and sit on the edge of it, lifting your bottom a few inches off the ground. As it gets easier, gradually have fewer and fewer folds of blanket underneath you, until you are ready to sit on the floor.

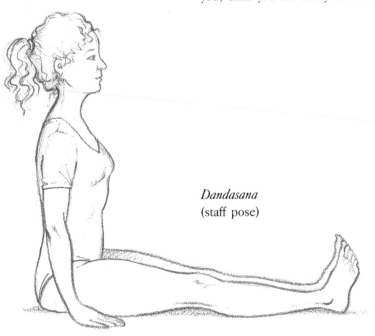

Dandasana
(staff pose)

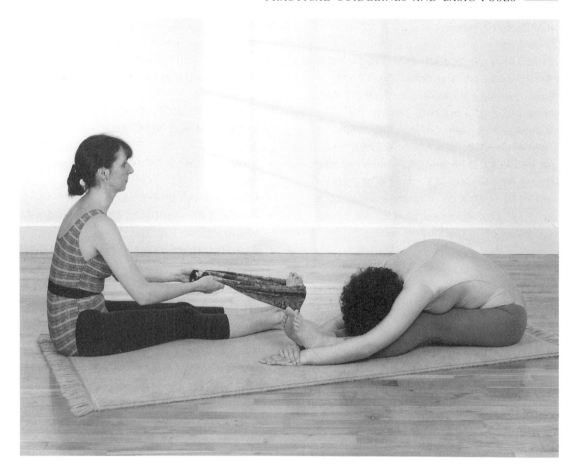

Paschimottanasana (strong forward stretch) and modified *paschimottanasana* with scarf

PASCHIMOTTANASANA – STRONG FORWARD STRETCH

- Sit in *dandasana*.
- On an exhalation, slide your hands down the outsides of your legs to your comfortable maximum without rounding your shoulders. Think of going forwards, not downwards.
- Inhale again, lifting your head, and stretching your spine and exhaling, stretch forwards a little more, and relax your head and neck.
- Breathe steadily and keep your face and throat relaxed. Stay as long as is comfortable for you.
- When you are ready to come out of the pose, inhale and lift your head, exhale and sit back up into *dandasana*.

VARIATION

If it is very difficult at first to make any forwards movement, loop a scarf or a belt around your feet and pull steadily on it to help yourself loosen up. Be careful not to round down and constrict your abdomen. At first *paschimottanasana* is a most frustrating posture.

It feels as though the backs of your legs will

never become supple and the swivelling forward movement in your hips will never come. Do not lose heart. I used to loathe this posture because it was uncomfortable and filled me with a sense of failure. Now I look forward to it as a luxurious stretch. Just keep doing it, and little by little the impossible will happen. One day, to your amazement, you will find yourself lying comfortably along the tops of your thighs. The whole of the back of your body from heels to head, is stretched in the pose. The abdominal muscles are toned and massaged in this posture too.

UPAVISTHA KONASANA – WIDE ANGLE STRETCH

- Sit in *dandasana*.
- Stretch your legs as wide apart as you can without tipping back onto your tailbone.
- Lift up through your spine, keeping the back of your neck long.
- Open your chest and release your shoulders.

- Place the backs of your hands on the fronts of your knees.
- Point your toes up to the ceiling.
- Breathe steadily with your face and throat relaxed.

Now add a forward bend.

- Move your hands to the floor in front of you.
- Inhale, sit well up out of your hips.
- Exhale, walk your hands forward and draw your body forwards and down.
- At your comfortable maximum, relax your head and neck. Breathe steadily.
- When you are ready to finish the pose, inhale and lift your head, exhale and walk your hands towards you to come up.

It does not matter if you can only go a couple of inches forwards at first. Your body stretches and opens gradually at its own best pace. One day you will find you are lying comfortably with your chest on the floor.

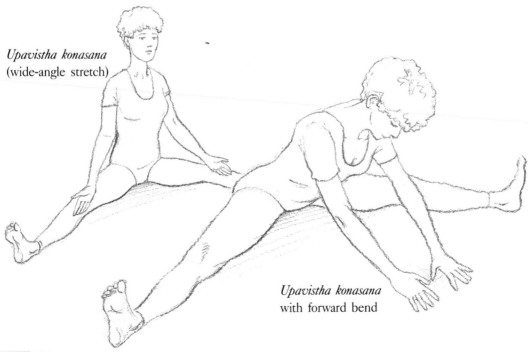

Upavistha konasana (wide-angle stretch)

Upavistha konasana with forward bend

BADDHA KONASANA – COBBLER POSE

- Sit in *dandasana*.
- Bring the soles of your feet together, then move them as close in towards the perineum as you can.
- Interlink your fingers and cup them round your feet.
- Let your knees fall as far to the floor as you can without falling back onto your tailbone.
- Lift spine and abdomen, open chest and release shoulders.
- Breathe steadily, keeping your face and throat relaxed.
- When you want to come out of the pose, lift your knees up with your hands, and stretch your legs out in front of you.

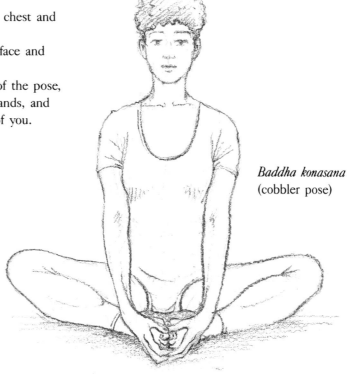

Baddha konasana
(cobbler pose)

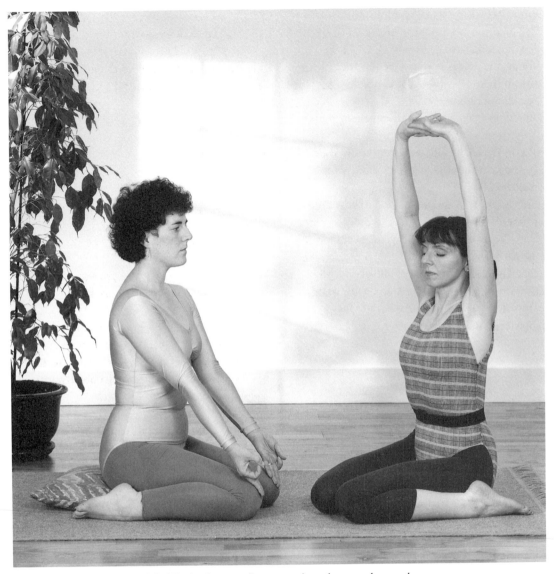

Modified *virasana* (hero pose) and upward stretch

VIRASANA – HERO POSE

Virasana gives a pleasing counter-movement to the wide abduction of the thighs in *upavistha* and *baddha konasana*. Many women enjoy sitting in this position naturally anyway, and are surprised to find that it is a yoga pose!

- Kneel up with your knees together and feet apart.

- Slowly, sit down between your feet.
- Interlink your fingers and inhale.
- As you exhale, push your hands out in front, palms away from you, then lift your arms vertically so that your palms face the ceiling.
- Release your shoulders, and relax your face and throat.
- Lift spine and abdomen and open your

chest, breathing steadily.

- When you want to come out of the pose, float your hands down into your lap and stretch your legs out in front of you. Gently massage your knees in a circular, stroking motion.

VARIATION

If it is impossible to sit down between your feet, place a couple of cushions, or your blanket, folded into a firm rectangular lift, behind you. Decrease the height of the 'lift' as your knees and hips become more flexible.

Virasana is the pose of the hero. This posture provides a good chance to remember and celebrate any strong, heroic women by whom we have been inspired, and also to acknowledge the heroism of our own lives.

Modified *virasana supta*

VIRASANA SUPTA -- RECLINING HERO POSE
After the upward stretch, try lying back in *virasana supta*. Until you are accustomed to this stretch, arrange two or three large pillows or cushions behind you, and rest back onto these.

- Sit in *virasana*.
- Hold onto your feet.
- On an exhalation, sink back onto one elbow, then the other.
- Unwind your shoulders and head down onto the pillows.
- On your next exhalation, stretch your arms straight up behind you.
- To come up, reverse the process, pressing into your elbows to lift yourself.

When you are supple enough, you can lie straight down onto the floor in *virasana supta*. This posture gives a delightful stretch to the front surface of the body and tones the digestive organs.

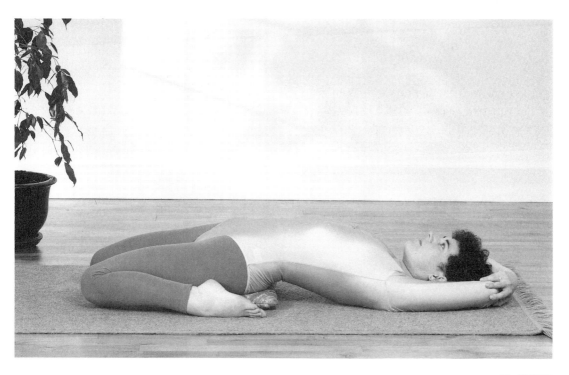

BHARADVAJASANA II – TWISTING POSE

- Sit in *dandasana*.
- Bring your left heel towards your perineum. If you can do so comfortably, lift it onto your right thigh in half lotus position.
- Bend your right knee, and tuck your right foot round behind you next to your hip – as in *virasana*, hero pose.
- When twisting, work from the base of the spine up. Exhaling, twist to your left, spiralling up from the root of the spine.
- Take the back of your right hand to the left of your left knee.
- Slide your left hand round behind your waist. Eventually you will hold the toes of your left foot.
- Turn and look over your right shoulder. Breathe steadily, face and throat soft.

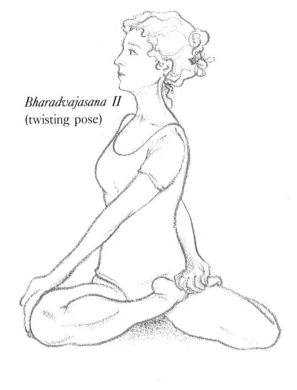

Bharadvajasana II
(twisting pose)

BENEFITS
This twisting action increases mobility in the spine and squeezes and massages the abdominal organs. The waist is toned and made more supple.

SALAMBA SARVANGASANA – SHOULDER STAND
The inverted postures of yoga give us a chance to enjoy being upside down again, as we did when we were children! Do not, however, practise inverted postures during a menstrual period. (There is a theoretical possibility of the flow being reversed and trickling back into the abdominal cavity.)

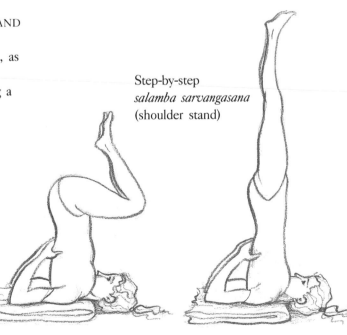

Step-by-step
salamba sarvangasana
(shoulder stand)

If you have not spent much time upside down since your childhood, approach the pose in easy stages, as in these illustrations. Once you are in comfortable balance in the shoulder stand, refine the pose by

- Lifting up through your spine.
- Making sure your legs stretch up vertically above your hips.
- Pushing your heels to the ceiling, elongating fully along the backs of your legs, then relax your feet so your toes are uppermost.
- Making sure your face, particularly your jaw, stays relaxed.

Twenty or thirty seconds will be long enough in this pose at first: gradually increase the time you spend there. When you want to come down, bend your knees and uncurl onto the floor, inch by inch. When your back is on the floor, place first one foot flat onto the ground, knee bent, then the other. Finally, slide your legs out straight. Think of your lower back spreading out. If you do feel a tightness there, slowly hug your knees back onto your chest again, and rock gently from side to side until all the discomfort is gone.

BENEFITS
Because of the chin lock in *salamba sarvangasana*, the thyroid and parathyroid glands are massaged. Constipation and headaches are relieved by this posture, and the legs are refreshed because pressure is taken off the valves in the veins. In fact *sarvanga* means 'the entire body', and this is a posture which is good for the whole body.

Awareness of Breathing

From birth till death we breathe, steadily and continuously – sleeping, waking, dreaming, still or moving. It is one of our ways of interacting and exchanging materials with the universe in which we live. Except at times of severe illness or emergency, this interaction takes place spontaneously, without any conscious effort on our part.

When we begin to do yoga postures we become aware of our breathing. We generally exhale as we stretch, inhale as we come up out of a stretch, and learn to breathe steadily and evenly even when in an intense stretch. Gradually the habit of exhalation on an effort, and continuing to breathe in a slow and steady rhythm even while under stress, spreads out into other parts of our lives. We learn to react to conflict or challenge not by a sharp intake of breath and clenched muscles, but with easy breathing and a strong, loose physical stance. Try these awareness exercises to extend your consciousness of your own breathing. There is a branch of yoga known as *pranayama*, connected with breathing awareness, but these awareness exercises are not really *pranayama* – *pranayama* is fundamentally to do with developing an awareness and control of *prana*, or life-energy, addressed through the movement and action of the breath.

ABDOMINAL BREATHING
This exercise helps to remind your body of the way you breathed deeply and easily as a little child – when your whole lungs filled and moved your diaphragm down so that your tummy expanded out when you breathed in, and deflated a little when you breathed out. Anxious adults often breathe only in the upper branches of their lungs, so that their abdomens suck in while they breathe in and their chests puff out; then as they breathe out, their abdomens sag forwards and their chests sink. See what your present pattern of breathing is, and whether this feels different.

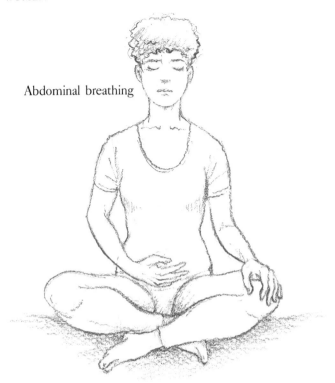

Abdominal breathing

- Sit with your legs comfortably crossed.
- Lift up tall out of your hips, keep the back of your neck long.
- Relax your shoulders.
- Rest your left hand on your left knee, rest your right hand on your abdomen below the navel.
- Begin to breathe a little more deeply, and a little more slowly than usual.
- When your rhythm is settled, breathe in through your nose, and out through your mouth.
- When this is happening fluently, take your attention to the hand on your abdomen. Direct the breath in down towards your hand, and draw the breath out up from behind your hand.
- When you have established a rhythm, make a tiny pause between each breath, so that you inhale and hesitate, then exhale and hesitate.

- Continue in your own rhythm. As you breathe in, you fill up and your abdomen swells a little. As you breathe out, you empty and your abdomen collapses a little.
- Keep your shoulders relaxed, your mouth and eyes relaxed.

When you have had a few minutes of this deep abdominal breathing, without disturbing yourself, take your right hand away from your abdomen and rest it on your right knee. Let your breathing return to an everyday level. When you are ready, blink your eyes open slowly to let in the light. Do not get up immediately – remain still for a few moments before you re-enter the activities of the day.

REVITALIZING BREATHING
This coordinated breathing and stretching exercise is a good way to revive flagging energies if you are feeling sluggish or low.

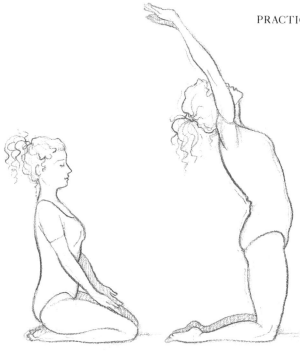

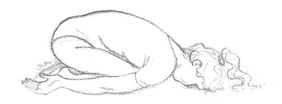

Three stages of revitalizing breathing exercise

- Begin by sitting on your heels, lifting your spine and abdomen, lengthening the back of your neck and spreading your chest and releasing your shoulders. Exhale.
- As you breathe in, kneel up, stretch your arms up, and stretch right up through from knees to fingertips.
- Exhale with a 'whooshing' noise through your mouth and stretch forwards and down. Lie on the top of your thighs, arms alongside your body.
- Repeat half a dozen times, then sit back on your heels again, tall and graceful, and feel the new energy in your body and mind.

If you ever feel dizzy doing this or any other breathing exercise, return straight away to everyday breathing. Work in every kind of yoga with a calm, alert observance, and you will not hurt yourself.

MEDITATION

Do not fear that meditation is an esoteric activity which you will probably not be able to do, or will certainly not be able to do properly. Meditation is not a strange activity; it is something we have all done spontaneously anyway, and the point of sometimes choosing to do it deliberately is to make this calming, healing and strengthening activity more a part of our lives.

During most of our waking hours our minds rattle around restlessly from one subject to another, one enthusiasm to another, one anxiety to another. Any time we become absorbed in an activity so that our mind is focused upon that one thing, we are freed from the kaleidoscope of outside distractions. We feel happy and peaceful at the time, and refreshed and revived afterwards. At other times we slip into a kind of spontaneous trance. You may gaze out of the train or bus

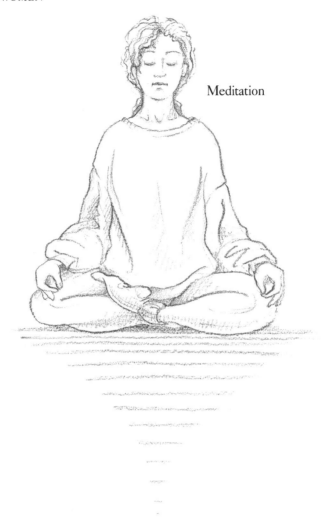

Meditation

window, and find with surprise that hours of the journey have passed while your mind has been in some other sphere. You may have sat gazing into the distance with your hands resting on your pregnant belly, feeling kicking and flickering baby movements under your hands, your thoughts 'miles away', or done familiar and mechanical work while your thoughts are free to clear, and float in unharassed free space. These are all examples of spontaneous meditative practices.

EXERCISE IN MEDITATION

- Sit comfortably, either cross-legged, or in half lotus pose. Lift and lengthen from the root of your spine to the crown of your head.
- Rest the backs of your hands on your knees. Join the thumb and index finger of each hand into a ring.
- Breathe in a slow, steady rhythm.
- Focus your mind on your mantra, *Om*, or an image such as a rose or a candle flame.

- As other thoughts intrude, simply observe them and let them go.

Four or five minutes will be long enough at first. You may be cross and restless initially, but bear with it. After a while, a feeling of calmness and steadiness will come.

Later on, you may be able to extend the length of time which you sit and let your mind become still. You will be able simply to 'stand back', to detach yourself from your mind and watch the flow of thoughts until they cease.

The effect of meditation is often illustrated with the metaphor of the lake. The true self is the bottom of the lake. The life of consciousness is the many metres of water above it. We stand on the shore trying to understand our true selves, but the surface of the water is constantly disturbed by pebbles and stones thrown into the water. These are our thoughts occurring. All we can see are the ripples and disturbances caused by the thoughts. Only by stopping the splashing of thoughts into the water can we let the surface settle. Then we are able to look through the clear water onto the deep bedrock at the bottom of the lake.

As with *savasana*, the effect is to put us more clearly in touch with our inner strength. Most women spend large stretches of their lives with multiple commitments, remembering myriad pieces of information, some factual, some about people's emotions and feelings, and coordinating them delicately. Like an air-traffic controller bringing many aircraft safely in to land, women negotiate the complexities of career and family life, caring for parents, partners, children, maintaining health and fitness of self and family members, catering, laundering, first-aiding, counselling, and being a social secretary. A short interlude of concentration or meditation at each yoga practice creates a wonderful sense of space in the self. Quietness spreads through body and mind, and another perspective on hectic schedules emerges, a slower, more detached, more consistent, bedrock self.

YANTRA AND MANDALA

Yantra and *mandala* are patterns which may be used for *tratak* or for continuous gazing and meditation. *Yantra* are usually geometrical in nature and tend to lead the eye in towards their centre, i.e. they are centripetal. *Mandala* may have a geometrical or a more fluid or organic look, and may contain representational pictures as well as patterns. They tend to lead the awareness to flow out from the centre and so their energy is centrifugal.

An upward pointing triangle in a *yantra* represents masculine energy, and a downward pointing triangle, feminine energy. They may sometimes be arranged on top of each other to make a star which represents harmony. A dot in the centre symbolizes the seed, the microcosm of potential. Circles in a *yantra* symbolize continuity – no beginning, no end, no dominance. Rectangular figures symbolize stability: the horizontal lines signifying repose, and the vertical lines signifying support. There may sometimes be stylized lotus petals included in a *yantra*, and sometimes a stylized rendering of the symbol for '*Om*'. The stillness of a *yantra* helps to settle and focus the mind.

Many natural organic structures are centrifugal like a *mandala*. Many flowers swirl or spread outwards like a *mandala*, the way cells are packed in a plant stem, as you would see them sectioned through a microscope, is a

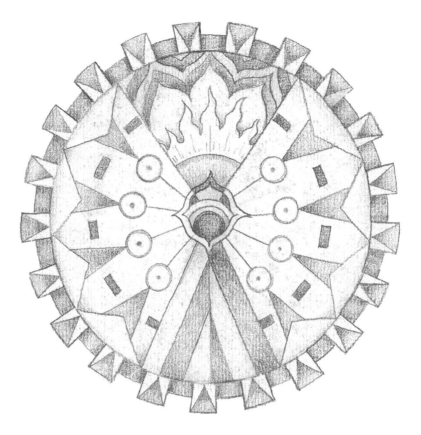

Yantra

mandala. The whorl of shells and shell fossils, the radiant effulgence around the sun setting among clouds, the earth itself, seen in all its innocent completeness from outer space by spacecraft, is a *mandala*.

The outward movement of energy in a *mandala* suggests a passage between different states – these can refer to general and cultural processes as well as private and inner ones. Movement, development and change, whatever those things represent to you at this particular moment, are elucidated by reflection on a *mandala*.

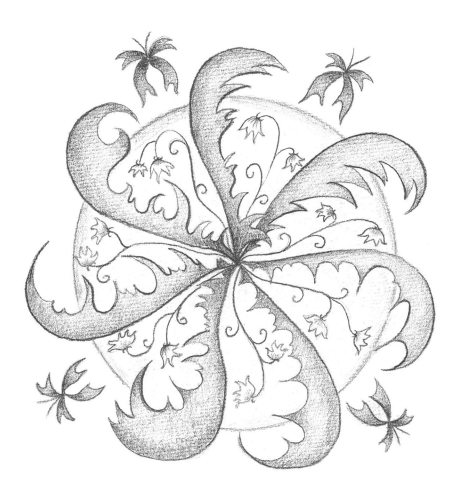

Mandala

CHAPTER THREE

LIFE PASSAGES

O ur lives as women are marked by a series of cycles and changes as our fertility evolves and varies and changes. Our bodies change in shape and texture, lightness, heaviness, different curves and volumes coming and going. Some women remain a fairly constant size and shape throughout their lives, while others wax and wane and alter profoundly with each decade. With the ebb and flow of different hormones we experience changes in our skin and hair, our ligaments and muscle tone. We become more or less vulnerable emotionally as the cycles evolve. We are sometimes bewildered by the range of body and character which seems to consitute the entity 'myself.'

Added to this we are surrounded daily by thousands of images presenting an ideal of woman as unscathed and unchanging, tall, thin, bronzed and athletic – as well as being thin she should also have the heavy swollen breasts of a lactating mother (so much for the collective unconscious of the tabloid press), and look passive and young. Women's magazines are deeply confused over this issue, publishing regular features about eating disorders, 'body facism' (the compulsion for everbody to undertake some sort of fitness régime), and accepting and loving one's body for what it is, while continuing to use models who reflect no such variety or broadness of vision, continuing to pile on the pressure for women to conform to one of these 'ideal' images.

Any woman who thinks about her body, its phases and changes, and her own views and emotions about it, may well find herself involved in a struggle with all kinds of contradictions. She may know that she feels confortable and healthy at one weight, but more powerful and sexual as she moves around in society at another, much lower, weight. She may have fantasies about radical/magical plastic surgery that would make her breasts bigger or smaller or change their shape, or carve layers away from hips or ankles. Few women escape the sense of having an 'unfavourite' part of their bodies. Few women contemplate the prospect of the changes age will bring without some misgivings.

Any woman who also sees herself as a rational person, or a feminist person, or someone committed to holistic thinking, will suffer, in addition to this, a sense of stupidity and guilt, as though she ought to be able simply to decide not to feel such things.

We are looking, perhaps, for a way to live with our physical bodies at their own comfortable, healthy sizes and shapes in all the range and variety which that implies, to be strong and fit and change and age with dignity and without denial. Yoga offers a medium through which those things can begin to happen. Because the body is strengthened, opened and challenged by the postures in an appropriate way, it becomes, as it were, *more* itself, more characteristic of itself, more true to itself. The sense of tuning into a deeper level of self which develops through centring at the beginning of a practice, through the practise of *savasana* (corpse or relaxation pose), and through spending time in concentration and meditation, can be a very steadying element when there is a great deal of physical and emotional fluctuation on the surface of our lives. It may be that the steady feeling has to do with containing an unchanging core in the centre of ourselves, or to do with an unchanging quality in the sense of peace itself.

If the phase of womanhood which you are going through feels important to you at the moment, you may like to build a yoga programme with that in mind. Remember to evolve a programme which begins with some calm time to come to centre, and ends with plenty of time with *savasana*. In the standing part of your programme include postures with strong forward and sideways stretches, and a balance to align your central upward strength. Include some appropriate back bends, sitting postures with the legs straight in front, with the legs stretched apart, and with the thighs rotated the other way (hero pose, page 26, and related postures). Programme in at least one of the many twists and, if appropriate, an upside down posture as well. You may want to do some breathing exercises, and some work with meditation too. *Savasana* closes your practice.

The poses in this chapter may feel useful to

illustrate and explore various life passages. Weave them into the basic shape of your programme if they attract you. Choose intuitively, be ready to reject anything that looks and feels too stressful or in any way awkward in relation to the way your body feels, and to choose anything, from whatever section, that seems to contain a movement, an expansion, or a mood that you need. Use the whole chapter as a resource to increase your vocabulary of asanas and as a stimulus to thinking more about what each posture means to and does for you.

Remember that these postures are not compulsory, nor are they a complete programme; they must be integrated into a full and balanced programme. Choose carefully and responsibly for yourself.

ADOLESCENCE

Somewhere between eight and sixteen years of age, the body of a little girl metamorphoses into that of a young woman. The date of the menarche (the beginning of menstrual periods) gets steadily younger and younger in the modern West. This seems to be linked with high levels of nutrition, and some research has also linked it with our extensive use of artifical light in the evenings: apparently one of the triggers for the release of hormones is the numbers of hours of light that have been experienced.

This presents girls who are very young in social terms, with the task of coping with periods, with their own sexuality, and with other people's reactions to it.

In a matter of months they may change completely in body shape from the straight, lithe lines of a little girl, to the curves and heavier volumes of maturity. While the monthly cycle of hormonal changes settles down, there is a tendency towards the moodiness and rawness which adults find so exasperating. The adolescent person finds it exasperating too. Once we have left adolescence behind, we are extremely insulting about it – describing someone's behaviour or emotions as 'adolescent' is almost always a put-down. This is hardly fair, and perhaps comes from one's own unresolved adolescent conflicts, still unexpectedly present during every other phase of our lives. One confidently expects on arriving at one's twenties or at the latest thirties, to be adult, competent and mature, and is shocked to find that in many respects one has not changed much since one was seventeen. Perhaps this is part of the strong reaction against all things 'adolescent'.

Practise of yoga can certainly help the condition of skin and hair, the steadying of moods and the steadying of the menstrual cycle. It can also provide a way of becoming more familiar with, and sensitive to, new body shapes, new axes and new strengths.

You may like to include these three poses in your practice.

HANUMANASANA – MONKEY POSE

Hanuman is the name of a strong and powerful monkey. He leapt across the sea with a huge stride, bringing healing herbs to a dying warrior. This pose represents the leap of *Hanuman*.

- Start by warming up the fronts of your thighs – right knee bent, foot on the floor between your hands, left leg straight out behind you. Then do the same stretch with left foot forwards, right leg straight out behind.
- Next, begin again with your right foot on the floor between your hands.
- Slide your left leg and top of your instep towards the floor, as far behind you as you can.

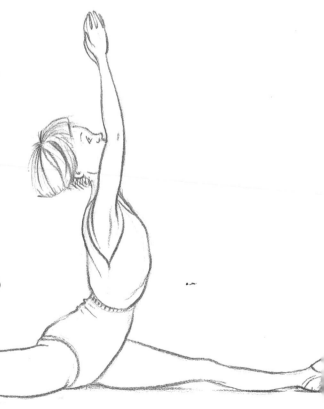

Hanumanasana (monkey pose) with arms overhead

- Keeping your weight in your hands, stretch your right leg out in front pushing your heel away.
- Go to your comfortable maximum. Keep your spine erect, your face soft and your shoulders relaxed.
- Remain for as long as feels right for you, breathing steadily. When you want to come out of the posture, pull your front leg back slowly.
- Repeat the stretch, with equal effort and attention, with the right foot in front.

When you can sit without stress in *hanumanasana* try bringing your hands together in front of your chest in *namaste*. When that is easy, stretch both arms up and join your palms high above your head. Do not let your shoulders hunch up.

Bring lightness and life to the pose by visualizing the leap. You have probably seen dancers leap across the stage like this, as though they were flying. Try to bring that feeling into your body.

UTTANA PADASANA - POSE OF TRANQUILLITY

- Lie on your back on the floor, making sure your centre line is straight.
- Exhaling, arch your upper back and rest the crown of your head on the floor. Take two or three breaths in this position.
- On another exhalation, lift your straight legs to an angle of 45° to the floor. Raise your arms, palms together, parallel to your legs.
- Feel your abdomen is strong, and your chest is free and open. You are balancing on the crown of your head and your buttocks.
- Breathe steadily in this balance. When you want to finish, exhale and lower your arms and legs. Exhale again and lengthen your spine to lie flat.
- If your lower back feels tight, hug your knees to your chest and rock gently from side to side.

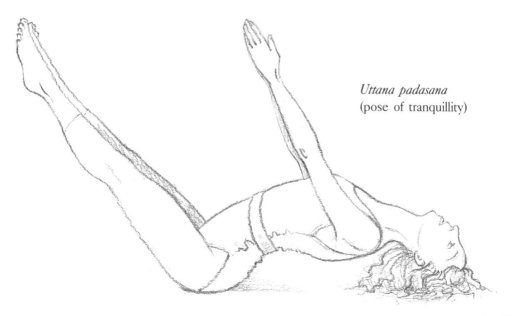

Uttana padasana
(pose of tranquillity)

VRSCHIKASANA – SCORPION POSE

The scorpion is an exciting pose which combines a back bend with a balance. It is pleasant to learn it when you are young and keep it in your 'vocabulary' as you grow older.

- Start learning this pose with the help of a friend, a blanket and a wall.
- Fold your blanket into a pad and place it next to the wall, to make a softer landing for your face if you should come down more quickly than you intend.
- Kneel on the floor facing the wall and rest your elbows on the floor, shoulder distance apart.
- Lay your forearms on the floor parallel to one another, with your fingers pointing forwards.
- Visualize your forearms as long 'feet' you are going to balance on.
- Hang your head forwards for a few seconds to lengthen and relax your neck and open your shoulders.
- Lift your head and move it forwards. Exhale, straighten your legs and stretch your hips in the air.
- On your first few attempts, simply try to straighten first one leg, then the other.
- Stretch one leg up and ask your friend to bring the foot to touch the wall. The other will naturally follow, and your friend can assist you to reach the wall with that too. Your friend can also help you to get down safely when you are ready.
- When you come down, sit back straight away into the praying stretch. You will eventually be able to move up and down into the pose without help, and rest just your toes on the wall, then work in free space.

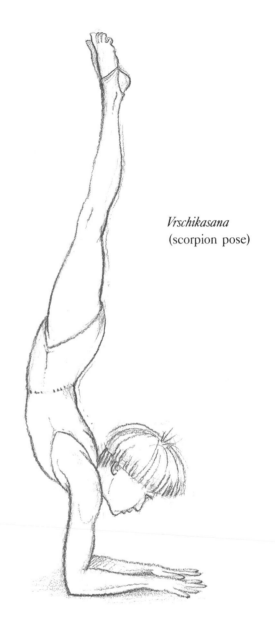

Vrschikasana
(scorpion pose)

MENSTRUAL CYCLE

The menstrual cycle generates an ebb and flow of hormones, an ebb and flow of energies and moods, throughout the fertile part of our life. Women who spend an extended time taking the contraceptive pill have a different kind of cycle, and may find it useful to be aware that when they stop the pill and fertile cycles begin again, they may find them surprisingly strong. One gradually becomes accustomed to them again, but at first they do feel very different.

The suppleness and strength from practising yoga help tremendously in flowing with the cycle rather than tensing up against it. Both posture and relaxation exercises also help with the cramps commonly experienced on the first couple of days of the period itself (but remember not to practise inverted postures during a period). In general, positive feelings about inhabiting your body and enjoying its functions make it more possible to move through this cyclic experience cheerfully. One need not attempt to pretend it is always pleasant, but it has its positive aspects. A sense of integration and concurrence with the natural world is also an important part of yoga: many of the postures are named after animals, plants, or natural objects like the mountains or the moon and in practising the pose you identify with that part of creation. Your growing awareness of your own physical structure and mass makes you feel more clearly part of the physical material of the universe, and less like an isolated organism in a world existing only like a technicolour movie in your own head. In those terms it is easier to feel and understand the repetitions of ovulation, fullness and bleeding.

These four postures may be useful for taking into your practice during menstruation, or the week before menstruation if that is a time when you feel full or bloated or very aware of your body in a different way, or any other time when your menstrual cycle is on your mind for any reason.

PADMASANA – LOTUS POSE

The lotus has its roots in the mud, its stem in the water and its beautiful flower in the sun. It reminds us that that is how we too can be – our roots are firmly in the mud, but we have the potential to flower out into the fresh air.

The quality of this pose is to have a steady, firmly spread base, open and uncongested hips and an upward lifting, free-breathing sensation in the upper body. The lotus flower is imagined where your halo would be (*sahasraha chakra* – see page 80). The pose helps to relieve swollen feelings in the pelvis and to lengthen the whole body which tends to contract forwards a little if you are either bloated or in pain. The steadiness of the base helps to 'ground' and stabilize the emotions.

- Sit in *dandasana*.
- Bend your right leg, and see if you can rest the top of your right instep on the top of your left thigh. If not, bring your right foot as close to your perineum as you can.
- Bend your left leg, and see if you can cross it on top of the right, laying the top of your left instep on the top of your right thigh. If you cannot do this yet, bring your left foot as close to the perineum as you can.
- Lift and align your spine, feel your hips open. Relax your shoulders.
- Rest your hands on your knees, or cup one inside another in your lap.
- Breathe steadily and think of the lotus.

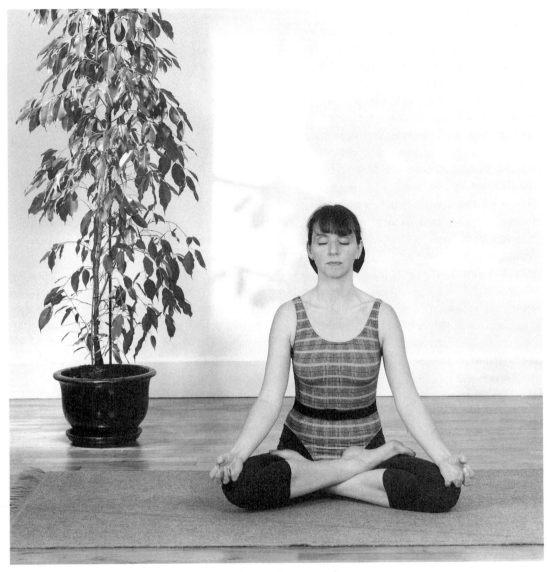

Padmasana (lotus pose)

- When you want to come out of the posture, untangle your legs carefully.
- Practise the pose with equal focus and attention, starting this time with your left leg.

If you have uncomfortable menstrual cramps, it is helpful to go into a forward bend from the full lotus position, so that your feet are pressing into the pelvic area, counteracting the tension of the cramp. If you cannot yet do full lotus, you can create the same effect by sitting cross-legged, make loose fists with your hands and rest them low down on the abdomen, and then stretch your upper body forwards and down – your fists will press into the area of the cramp and relax it somewhat.

URDHVA DHANURASANA – BRIDGE POSE

Urdhva dhanurasana is the position which, as children, we called 'crab'. It is a lovely posture for relieving bloated feelings in the abdomen, because it gives a long, strong stretch to the front of the body, while arching your spine in a powerful back bend. It also brings a sense of strength and confidence.

- Lie on your back with your knees bent and feet flat on the floor.
- Rest your hands on the floor bent back (fingers pointing towards your feet), at shoulder level.
- When you feel ready, come up onto the crown of your head.

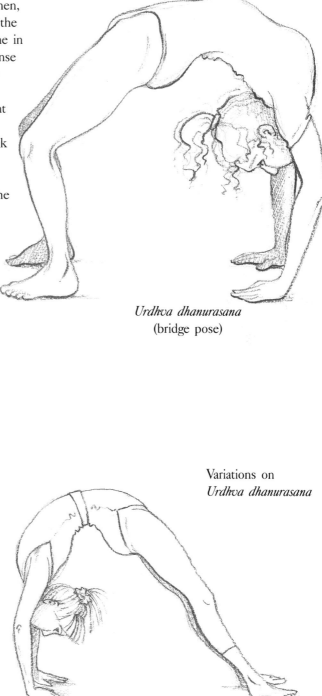

Urdhva dhanurasana
(bridge pose)

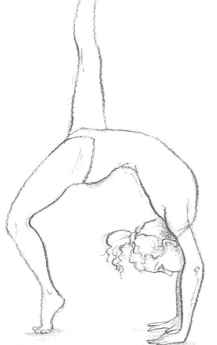

Variations on
Urdhva dhanurasana

- Next, exhale, and lift up onto hands and feet, arms and legs strong, breathing steadily.
- Remain for a few seconds – you can stay longer when you become stronger and more confident.
- When you want to come down, lift your head a little, and with your neck long, unwind your spine slowly and with control onto the floor.
- When your whole spine is on the floor, hug your knees onto your chest and rock slowly from side to side.

VARIATIONS

When *urdhva dhanurasana* becomes easy, you can try the variation shown on page 43.

ARDHA CHANDRASANA – HALF MOON POSE

People who work or travel at night, or live in the country away from artificial night lighting, become aware of the phases of the moon. We are missing out when we live a life when we no longer see the moon or know whether it is waxing, full, or waning. If you start to look out for the moon you can see where your own cycle fits with that of the moon.

Many diaries have a menstrual calendar which will show how your particular rhythm ripples across the months.

The half moon pose is triangle pose *trikonasana*, extended out into a balance. You can try it first with your back against a wall for support, and progress to performing the pose in free space.

- Inhale and lay your upper arm along the top edge of your waist.
- Exhale, bend the front knee, take your front hand to the floor 12 inches ahead of your front foot, and lift and straighten the back leg parallel to the floor.

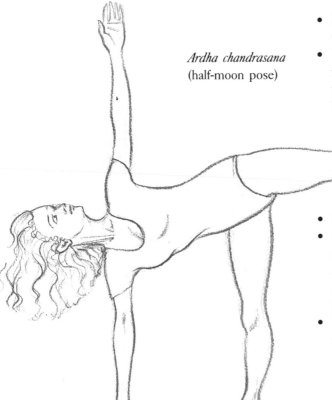

Ardha chandrasana (half-moon pose)

- Stretch the heel of the lifted leg away.
- Focus your gaze on something straight ahead. When you feel stable enough to do so, stretch your upper arm up into the air, palm forwards. Breathe steadily, keeping your face and throat relaxed.
- To come down, return to *trikonasana*, then come up in the usual way.

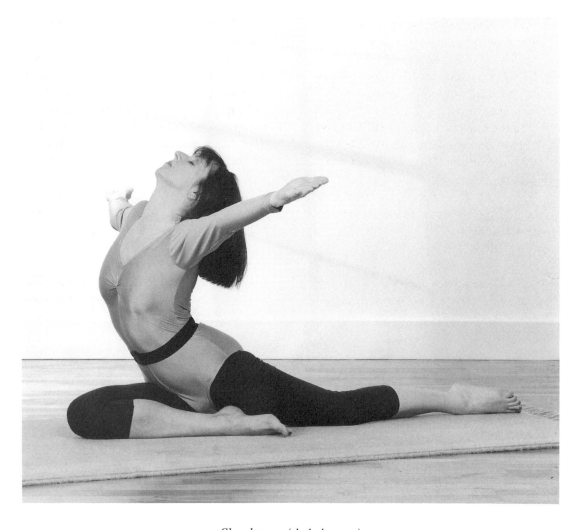

Chatakasana (skylark pose)

CHATAKASANA - SKYLARK POSE
This beautiful pose gives a feeling of lightness
– a marvellous way to balance any sense of
sluggishness or heaviness. If you have
practised *hanumanasana* you will not find it
difficult.

- Begin with your hands on the floor, hip
distance apart, your right knee bent and
your right foot between your hands.
- Ease your left leg out behind you, the top
of your instep on the floor, knee facing

down. Be careful that your back leg is
aligned straight, and not veering to left or
right.
- Bring your bent right knee to the ground
and tuck your right foot into your
perineum. Balance with your fingertips on
the floor on either side of your hips.
- As you exhale, stretch your arms out,
palms up, behind you, and stretch your
spine up and back. Breathe steadily.
- When you want to come out of the
posture, exhale and come into a cross-

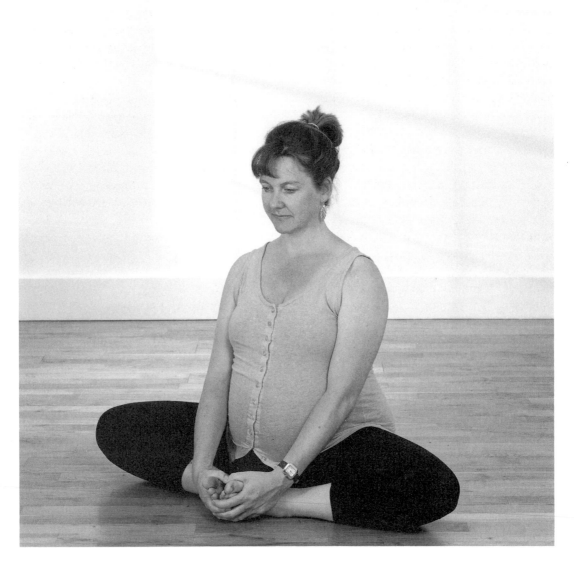

Baddha konasana (cobbler pose) in eighth month of pregnancy

legged position until your breathing and
heartbeat have settled.
• Then do *chatakasana* with equal focus and
attention, this time with the other leg in
front.

PREGNANCY

During the first three months of an
uncomplicated pregnancy you can
practise all your normal postures as the baby
is still tucked down into your pelvis. However,
if you do ever feel stressed, come gently out
of the posture and rest in *savasana* or lie on

your side until you feel comfortable again. If you have had bleeding or any other difficulties, discuss with your midwife when it would be safe and advisable for you to begin doing yoga again. Take your yoga book with you to show your midwife the stretches you would like to do if you think she may not be familiar with yoga poses.

After twelve weeks or so you will feel the fundus (the top of the uterus) gradually rising up into the abdomen. There are a few postures which should be avoided once this starts to happen: firstly anything which involves lying on your tummy on the floor (such as cobra, or locust); secondly, strong back bends (like *urdhva dhanurasana* and, unless you are very confident in it, *ustrasana*), and any twisting postures which make your abdomen feel squashed. Unless you have practised for several years, or are working with an experienced teacher, avoid inverted postures, by doing dog pose (no. 8 in *surya namaskar*, page 69) and modified headstand (head and arms in position, hips up, feet on floor) instead.

Be attentive to your body and avoid anything which feels forced or wrong. As your abdomen grows, be aware that your centre of gravity will change and your balance will be different, particularly in poses like *trikonasana*.

The joy of yoga in pregnancy is the opportunity to enjoy your changing shape and swelling curves, while remaining graceful and powerful. The stretching and mobility help to relieve back and shoulder aches, and to expand and strengthen the pelvic outlet and the pelvic floor. Both *savasana* and meditation are a chance to reflect on the miracle of the small life gradually growing to independence inside you.

SQUATTING POSE
This comfortable and relaxing posture becomes alien to us when we sit on chairs and wear high-heeled shoes, and we lose the lovely opening and flexibility in our hips.

• Stand with your feet 2–2½ feet apart, toes turned out.

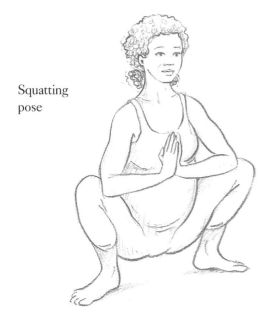

Squatting
pose

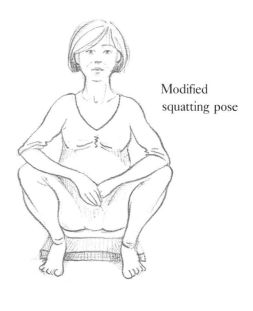

Modified
squatting pose

- Put your hands palm to palm together in front of you in *namaste*.
- As you exhale, squat down, slide your elbows inside your knees, lift your spine and relax your shoulders.
- Breathe steadily, keep your face and throat soft.
- To come out of the posture, either exhale, push into your feet and stand up, or sit gently down and straighten your legs.

VARIATION

You may need to relearn squatting with your heels resting on a thick book (a dictionary or a phone book would be useful) and your elbows resting loosely on your knees.

Gradually decrease the height of the lift under your heels as the weeks go by, and you will eventually find your heels resting comfortably on the floor. When you can, ease your elbows between your knees and press your palms together, levering your thighs wider apart.

FROG POSE AND PELVIC FLOOR EXERCISE

- Kneel with your feet together and knees apart.
- On an exhalation sit your bottom back onto your heels, or as far back as you comfortably can.

- Walk your hands as far forwards along the floor as you can, making the front and the back of your body as long as you can.
- Breathe steadily, with your face and throat relaxed.
- When you want to come out of the posture, walk your hands towards you on an inhalation and sit up.

When you have extended into the pose of the frog, focus on your pelvic floor muscles. If you aren't sure where these are, imagine that you need to go to the toilet, but that there is no toilet available nearby. Contract the muscles that you would need to contract in that situation – a ring of muscles around the front passage, and another ring around the back passage, arranged together like a figure of eight. At first you may find you can hardly cause the muscles to contract voluntarily at all, but it is very important to learn to strengthen these muscles, so persevere.

Squeeze and release your pelvic floor muscles half a dozen times when you are in the frog pose, then breathe in and lift your head, exhale and walk your hands towards you to come up.

Frog pose opens the hips and thighs, and also gives a sense of stretching and opening to the lower back which helps to alleviate the tender

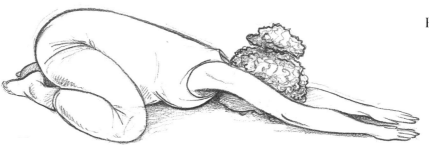

Frog pose

backache that arises because of the softening of ligaments caused by hormonal changes. This softening will often make your poses more open and extended during pregnancy, and you will find that so long as you practise fairly steadily, you can carry that extra stretch and movement with you when the pregnancy is over. The softening does, however, mean that you should treat your joints with extra respect and, particularly, never be tempted to bounce limbs or joints in order to increase your stretch.

When you kneel or stand up, take your thoughts once more to your pelvic floor muscles. You will observe that they are in roughly the area that a sanitary towel would cover. Think about what they are doing and you will realize, once you are vertical, that they are what hold your insides in! During pregnancy they also hold in several pounds of baby, placenta, liquor and membranes as well.

Clearly it is important to keep these muscles in good condition, and doing so will help to prevent incontinence and prolapse later on. On the positive side, once you are aware of and in touch with these muscles, you will be more able to release and relax them when the baby is born, and your vaginal muscle tone will improve more quickly after the birth. Every time it crosses your mind, squeeze and release your pelvic floor half a dozen times.

ANJANEYASANA – CRESCENT MOON POSE

When it is no longer possible to get down onto your tummy and practise cobra, you will probably find yourself longing for a good back bend. *Anjaneyasana*, in a modified version as in the illustration, may provide you with one.

- Kneel with your left knee on the floor and your right foot on the floor with your right knee bent.
- Make sure your body is facing fully to the

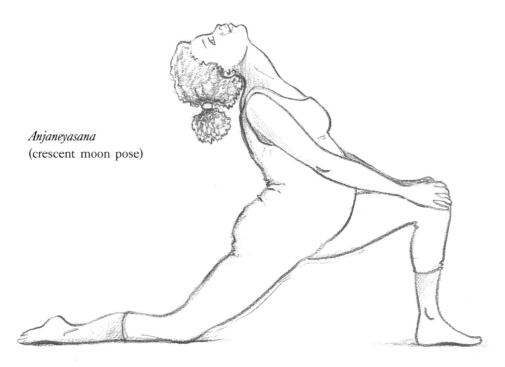

Anjaneyasana
(crescent moon pose)

front, and not turned at an angle.

- Place your hands on your front knee to steady yourself.
- Stretch your left leg further back, stretching the front of your thigh.
- On an exhalation, grow taller, and then bend your lengthened spine backwards.
- When you want to come out of the pose, inhale and lift your head, and exhaling, come up.
- Rest in frog pose.
- When you have had a rest, repeat *anjaneyasana*, with equal effort and focus, with the other leg in front.

ABDOMINAL BREATHING AND MODIFIED
SAVASANA

Abdominal breathing as described in Chapter 2 (pages 29–30) is an invaluable way of calming down during pregnancy. This steady breath combined, when it becomes necessary, with a swaying movement of the hips, in any position where your hips are relaxed and open and your torso is inclined forwards in relation to your hips (this helps to open your pelvis), can help to carry you through your contractions in the first stage of labour.

In the later months of pregnancy, if you become heavy and weary, you may like to practise both abdominal breathing and *savasana*, lying on your side.

Choose your left side, because then your heavy uterus is not pressing onto your vena cava, the major vessel returning blood to your heart. The vena cava runs along the right-hand side of the spinal column, so by lying on the left side, you are rolling the weight of the uterus away from it. Have a cushion or pillow under your head, and another under your bent right knee, and make your arms comfortable either by sliding your left arm out under you to your left side, or if your breasts

are too sore for this, by curling your arms loosely into a foetal position, keeping your shoulders and chest as loose and open as you can.

Do a few cycles of abdominal breathing, then allow your breath to settle where it wants to: it will probably be slow and light. Now rest in *savasana*, muscles and joints heavy and soft, face and throat soft, back soft and spreading out, feet and hands warm and heavy.

After some time in *savasana* you may feel you want to put a hand onto your abdomen and say hello to the baby.

The baby may sometimes swim over and push back onto your hand! This pre-birth communication comes naturally to many mothers and many babies, and is a happy beginning to your relationship with one another.

Remember that the poses suggested here are not a complete sequence for pregnancy, but should be fitted into a full and balanced programme as we have described. Do not hesitate to redesign your programme every 5 or 6 weeks during pregnancy to reflect your body's different shape and different needs, and do not be afraid to concentrate more on the sitting poses in the last few weeks if you are tired. Sometimes our modern culture's dictum that, as a woman, you should be fit, thin, and sexually available every moment of your life leaves your ability to work out how you feel and what you want (let alone how to get it) in shreds. Is it lazy, will you be gross and slothful if you only or primarily do floor poses in the last weeks of pregnancy? Of course not. What is right for you today? Choose that. Do not feel inadequate if you are not sure what it is – most of our conditioning and education has prompted us to think that what our own impulse is will probably be wrong. Just sit with it until it becomes clear to you what it is. Do not be afraid to be sometimes large and sometimes small, to be sometimes strong and sometimes weak, sometimes fast and sometimes slow.

To every thing there is a season, and a time to every purpose under the heaven:
A time to be born, and a time to die; a time to plant, and a time to pluck up that which is planted;
A time to kill, and a time to heal; a time to break down and a time to build up;
A time to weep and a time to laugh; a time to mourn and a time to dance; . . .
A time to get and a time to lose, a time to keep and a time to cast away; . . .
A time to love, and a time to hate; a time of war, and a time of peace . . .
Ecclesiastes 3:1

This is echoed in Lao Tzu:

For all things there is a time for going ahead, and a time for following behind,
A time for slow breathing, and a time for fast breathing,
A time to grow in strength and a time to decay,
A time to be up and a time to be down.
Therefore the sage avoids all extremes, excesses, and extravagances.

Not every woman is or should be an athlete right through her pregnancy. What we can do for each other is to accept and celebrate the whole spectrum of shape, fitness and frame of mind in each of us at this special time.

THE POST-NATAL MONTHS

Psychologists tell us that new mothers are involved in something called 'primary preoccupation' with their babies. New mothers of course know that their primary preoccupation is with getting enough sleep! Actually, of course the involvement with the new baby is, in turns, exciting, heartrendingly tender, tedious, frustrating, delightful, all manner of contradictory qualities simultaneously and this is, therefore, a demanding time for the mother. Many of us undertake, without the support of an extended family, the months of learning to live with a new, and initially very dependent little person, often with little sleep and a cut in income and social recognition. (For all the lip service our society pays to 'family values', women caring for children are often, astonishingly, described as 'not working'.) We are also, perhaps, learning the art of breastfeeding, trying to work out a new identity for ourselves and trying to rest, heal and restrengthen our bodies.

Many women are preoccupied, too, with when they might be able to get back into their ordinary clothes again, and the change from the magnificent fullness of 9 months of pregnancy, to a shape which is much larger than you were before you became pregnant, can be a great shock. Patience is really the answer. If you are not one of the (very few) women who revert immediately to their pre-pregnant shape, do not panic and do not hate your body. Its capacity for change and recovery is tremendous, and you can be well-toned and have a defined shape again, it simply takes time. (One woman, who always looked pretty slim to me, confided, 'It was 16 weeks after the birth before I could get my jeans past my *knees*.')

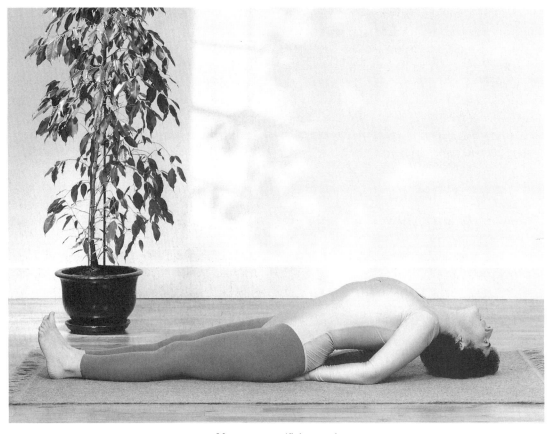

Matsayasana (fish pose)

You can begin doing postures gently any time you feel like it 2 weeks after the delivery. (If you had a Caesarean section you will want to leave it a few weeks longer.) Do not do inverted postures while you are still losing lochia (the post-natal bleeding). If you notice that your bleeding gets heavier during or after doing postures, or indeed during or after any activity, it indicates that you are overdoing things, and should rest more.

Begin by attempting perhaps five or six postures at the most a day, and gradually increase the length of the programme during the following weeks, as you grow stronger.

Good quality rest during the weeks after the

birth of a baby is more valuable than money in the bank. At any interlude or opportunity, have a few minutes of *savasana*, or abdominal breathing, or quiet meditation. You can conserve energy and reach your deep inner core of strength by doing so.

You will enjoy your new lightness when you remake your programme again, though do watch your balance in the standing poses, as your centre of gravity is, yet again, different from how it was before the baby was born. You may like to incorporate some of these postures into your programme. Go gently, the hormones which loosened your ligaments and joints during pregnancy may still be circulating in your body up to six months after the birth.

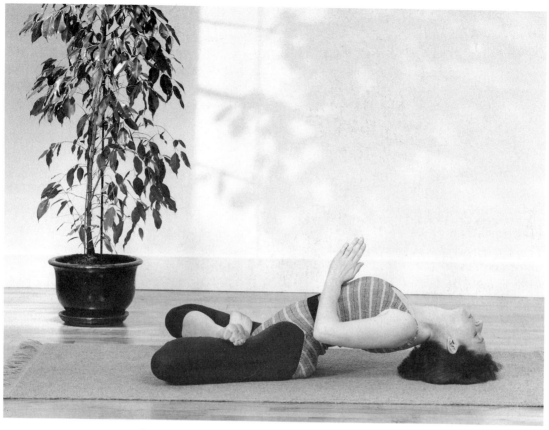

Matsayasana in *padmasana* (fish pose in lotus pose)

MATSAYASANA – FISH POSE

This pose can come into your practice as a back bend. It is also a useful counter-posture to follow a shoulder stand, taking any residual tension out of neck and shoulders.

- Lie on your back, ensuring that your centre line is straight.
- Place your hands palms down, under your hips.
- On an exhalation, press your elbows into the ground, arch your upper back, and come up onto the crown of your head.
- Lengthen all along your legs and stretch your heels away.
- Breathe steadily, keep your chest open and your shoulders soft.

- To come out of the pose, lift your head gently, then lay it on the ground, slide your arms out from underneath you and rest.

VARIATION

If you are comfortable in *padmasana*, lotus pose, move into *matsayasana* by leaning back on your elbows, then bring the crown of your head to the floor. Press your palms together above your heart.

Janu sirsasana
(seated forward stretch)

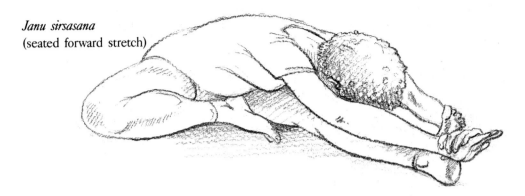

JANU SIRSASANA – SEATED FORWARD
STRETCH
This can be included as a forward bend.

- Sit in *dandasana*.
- Bring your left heel into your perineum and open your left hip and knee out to the side.
- Inhale and stretch up out of your hips, stretch both arms straight up in the air.

- As you exhale, stretch forwards and then down along the straight leg, holding onto your leg or foot at your own comfortable maximum.
- Relax your head and neck. Keep your back flat – the bend is from the top of the thigh, not the back of the waist. Breathe steadily and relax your face and throat.
- To come up, exhale and sit up into *dandasana*.
- Do the posture again with just as much care with the other leg bent.

ANANTASANA – WHEEL POSE
Anantasana is named after the serpent from whose centre the lotus grew. It represents the wheel of creativity. It is an appropriate pose for this moment in your life. You have joined in creating a new baby, you are engaged in creating a new family, and you are also creating a new identity and place in the world for yourself. This is apart from perhaps creating breast milk, a constant stream of meals and laundry and a pleasant environment for your family, on top of any other projects you might have.

Anantasana
(wheel pose)

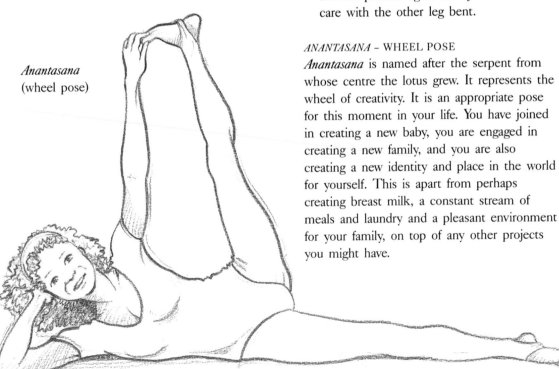

Anantasana is a combination between a tricky balance and an intense stretch – as a new mother you are familiar with the feeling!

It also helps to maintain the extra stretch and openness of hips and thighs which you will have developed if you practised yoga during your pregnancy.

- Lie on your side resting your head on your lower hand; check your alignment.
- Focus your gaze to enhance your balance.
- Bend the knee of the upper leg. Link two fingers of the upper hand round the big toe of the upper foot.
- As you exhale, straighten the upper leg.
- Breathe steadily. Keep your face serene.
- To come out of the posture, inhale and bend the upper leg, exhale and release your grip on the toe, and lay the top leg along the lower one again.

Have a rest, and then roll over onto your other side to do *anantasana* again, stretching up with the other leg this time.

THE MENOPAUSE

At any time between our late thirties and our early sixties we may find ourselves in the menopause, the phase which may last anything between a few months and a couple of years, during which we move through the last part of our fertility and into a new and different time.

The menopause has had a bad press for a long time, and certainly many of us find ourselves vulnerable and confused as the physiological changes gradually reach a new equilibrium within us. Nevertheless, our lives as women have taught us well how to adapt and cope with change, and how to make and remake our lives again and again as circumstances and focus change.

Women have begun to write, speak and share about the menopause, and these resources may be useful as we experience it. Many well woman centres and family planning clinics organize menopause groups where both the physical and emotional aspects can be discussed.

It is useful to continue with yoga – the physical activity helps us to retain muscle tone and flexibility, and to stimulate and regulate the workings of the soft inner organs. If you have practised yoga for a long time, your flexibility will be maintained. If you have only just made a beginning with yoga, work gently and remember always only to go to the right place for yourself in any of the stretches. Your body will soon feel loose and refreshed.

When menopause arises as a crisis for us it is sometimes not only the physical symptoms but also the predicament of being a woman undeniably ageing in a culture which seems only to value young women. One woman said, 'I felt marginalized as soon as I stopped being what could be very clearly classed as young and pretty.' We have a bad record of respecting and caring for any older people irrespective of gender in the modern West, so no wonder we feel apprehensive about it.

We may not be able to affect the whole culture immediately, but we can affect our own sense of ourselves, and other people's perception of us. We need to become attuned to the shape of our time on earth and accept the ageing process as inevitable and as having its own form and dignity. This does not mean becoming depressed and decrepit, but it does mean finding out how we want to feel, move and look, and not panicking when it has its own quality which is different from how we felt, moved and looked in our twenties. Our experiences may not all be happy but they are rich and varied, and give us a depth, and a capacity for compassion.

Look out for images – photographs, news pictures, paintings, sculptures, of strong older women being themselves without fear; these will inspire you.

These poses may be useful, fitted into your basic programme.

VIRABHADRASANA – WARRIOR POSE I

Virabhadrasana I is the first form of the warrior pose. It brings a feeling of power and strength. Use this pose as a chance to celebrate your personal battles and your own courage.

- Stand in *tadasana*.
- Step your feet 4–4½ feet apart. Turn your left foot in and your right foot out, right heel in line with left instep.
- Put your hands palm to palm together in front of your heart, in *namaste*.
- On an exhalation, turn your hips and chest to face in the direction of your right leg.
- Inhale again. As you exhale, bend your front knee so your shin stays vertical and your thigh is parallel to the floor.
- Breathe steadily. Take your weight down onto the outside of your back foot.
- When you are ready, on an inhalation, straighten the front knee. Turn your feet the other way, and do *virabhadrasana I* bending the other leg, just as accurately and carefully.

VARIATION

Practise *virabhadrasana* with your arms stretched straight up, palms facing each other. This makes the pose even more vigorous and should *not* be done during pregnancy or if you have high blood pressure.

DRAGONFLY POSE

The pose of the dragonfly is a charming pose to look at and a pleasant one to perform. The lower back is stretched and the abdomen and thighs are stretched and extended. The shoulders are working too in the completed pose. Approach the pose of the dragonfly one step at a time and do not force your body to go farther than it is ready to.

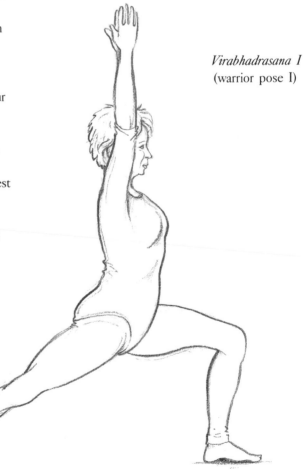

Virabhadrasana I
(warrior pose I)

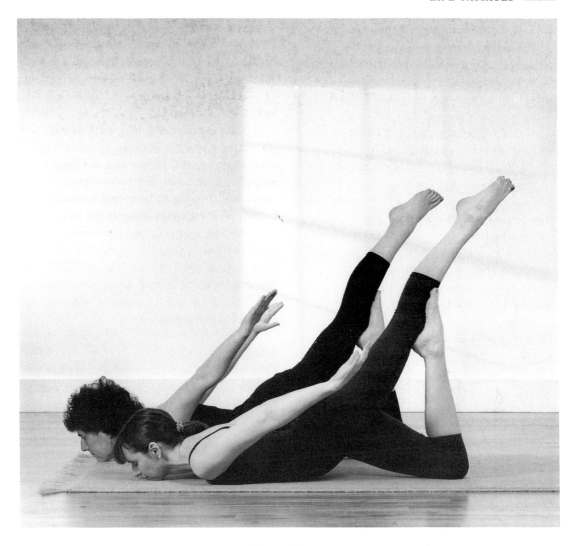

Dragonfly pose

- Lie on the floor on your front. Ensure your centre line is straight.
- Slide your hands, palms upwards, under the fronts of your thighs to stabilize yourself.
- Bring your forehead to the floor.
- Bend your right knee, exhale and lift your left leg, balancing your left knee on your right foot.
- Remain for a few seconds, breathing steadily, then exhaling, unbend your right leg and slowly lower.

- Push up onto all fours on an inhalation, and sit back in praying stretch on an exhalation.
- Let your heart rate and breathing return to normal, then lie down again and practise the pose carefully on the other side.

VARIATION
When you are used to dragonfly pose, intensify it by placing your chin on the ground and lifting straight arms up behind you.

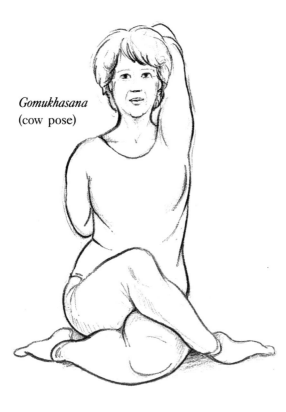

Gomukhasana
(cow pose)

GOMUKHASANA – COW POSE

- Sit in *dandasana*.
- Bend your left knee and tuck your left heel under your right buttock.
- Cross your right knee over and place it on top of your left knee.
- Centre and balance yourself, lifting your spine.
- Wriggle your right arm up between your shoulder blades.
- Inhale and stretch your left arm up. Exhale, bend the elbow, and reach down to catch your right hand with your left.
- Breathe steadily with your eyes soft and throat relaxed.
- To come out of the posture, inhale, release your fingers and stretch your left arm up,

exhale and float it down. Inhale again and as you exhale, untangle your legs.
- Repeat the pose, equally sensitively, to the other side.

VARIATIONS
It may be useful at first to place a folded blanket or a cushion between your heels and to sit back on that. If you cannot straight away link your hands behind you, hold a sock or scarf in your upper hand and catch the bottom of it with your lower hand. You will eventually be able to bring your hands together.

You may notice a striking asymmetry in this pose: that is all right – practising yoga will eventually even things up.

BENEFITS
Dragonfly pose and cow pose are excellent counter-balancing postures. Dragonfly brings lightness, flair and balance, and cow pose maintains flexibility in knees, hips and shoulders, as well as being very grounding and calming.

The menopause is not a rite of passage held in high regard in our Western urban culture. Instead of seeing it as an opportunity to move into detachment and wisdom, we panic (and this is not surprising in a youth-worshipping society) about the visible signs of ageing and are deeply confused as to what it means for our sexuality. To say that somebody is 'menopausal' is almost always an insult.

Yoga cannot rescue us from these confusions, but it can strengthen our bodies, calm our intellects, and sustain our spiritual selves while we struggle with them.

CHAPTER FOUR

LIFE EVENTS

The suggestions for this chapter concern choosing extra postures to bring into your basic programme when your life is passing through particular events or emotional phases. The reasons for choosing the poses mentioned here are partly physiological and partly interpretative. As with the postures in the *Life Passages* section, these are suggestions for you to use creatively yourself. Omit any which feel inappropriate for you, and choose any that feel right even if they do not appear to match specifically with the 'life event' you are experiencing now. There may, for example, be times when you feel very alone even though apparently surrounded by people, or times when you feel a failure even though on the surface of your life you seem to be in a successful phase. Of course, the paradox could be the other way around, and although the circumstances of your life look grim, you could be feeling a real satisfaction and sense of your own strength and success in survival.

Long practice of yoga makes a subtle alteration in our emotional perspective. It is described by Eknath Easwaran in his introduction to the *Bhagavad Gita* with a rather down-to-earth simile:

When I look at a fresh, ripe, mango, it is natural for my senses to respond; that is their nature. But I should be able to stand aside and watch this interaction with detachment, the way people stand and watch while movers unload a van. In that way I can enjoy what my senses report without ever having to act compulsively on their likes and dislikes.

The Bhagavad Gita; *page 26, trans. Easwaran, Arkana, 1988*

Because we value and admire passionate involvement and commitment in our culture, we may initially dislike the idea of detachment. However, a sense of what is meant by detachment grows in the context of yoga: it is not a cold indifference, more a sense of being both in and out of a situation simultaneously, of intense involvement balanced by a watching and observing in a kind of compassionate detachment. This shift of attitude develops spontaneously over the months and years that we practise.

Postures in this chapter, then, can be used for celebration or comfort, or whatever you feel you need.

ALONE OR SEPARATED

We may experience isolation at many times in our lives. It may come because we are socially or geographically isolated, or financially isolated – too broke to go out, or join classes, or participate in things. We may be working with colleagues who do not seem to be on our wavelength, or perhaps there are times when nobody in our immediate family is attending to anything we think, feel, or say.

Necessity may have separated us from loved friends or partners, or they may have rejected and abandoned us. This last is perhaps the most devastating of all. The particular impact on women of broken or damaged partnerships is well described by Jean Baker Miller in her book *Towards a New Psychology of Women*:

> . . . *women stay with, build on, and develop in a context of attachment to and affiliation with others. Indeed, women's sense of self* [*is*] *very much organized around being able to make and then maintain affiliation and relationships. Eventually for many women, the threat of disruption of an affiliation is perceived not as just a loss of a relationship but as something closer to a total loss of self* . . .

This feeling can come too, when a loved friend or partner dies. Thus, when we lose a loving partnership we are faced not only with remaking our lives, but, at a fundamental level, with remaking ourselves. Although it is a struggle, if you are in the middle of this at the moment, try to hold on to the fact that it is possible and will eventually happen that, although you can be bruised and miserable, the central and unique quality that makes you yourself cannot be dismantled:

> *The Self cannot be pierced by weapons or burned by fire; water cannot wet it, nor can the wind dry it. It is everlasting and infinite, standing on the motionless foundations of eternity.*
>
> Bhagavad Gita *2:23, 24, trans. Easwaran, Arkana, 1988*

'Self' here does not mean what we call 'ego', but is closer to what we might call 'soul' or 'spirit'. This is not to suggest that the pain we feel is not real and vivid, but that there is a part of ourselves that cannot be destroyed.

Sometimes we are happy to be alone, and love the sense of clarity and independence which a chosen and powerful independence brings. If parts of our life have been overcrowded we may seek out and exult in times to move freely about the world, think our own thoughts through to the end and become more familiar with our own moods and rhythms, away from the necessity of adapting to others.

TADASANA – MOUNTAIN POSE
(See page 8)
Whether or not you are alone or feeling alone by choice, and whether or not you feel positive about it, *tadasana* is an important posture.

Spend time really rooting down from beneath the soles of your feet well into the earth. Grow up through your spine and feel the crown of your head aspiring towards the sky. Feel the strength in your legs.

If you are enjoying your solitude, it can be exhilarating to visualize yourself standing in *tadasana* from gradually further and further away, until you seem to see yourself as a tiny figure standing on the curved surface of the planet. You are alone but also part of the world, the Gaia organism, standing on the skin of the beautiful earth.

If you feel lonely, sense what is happening in your body. It may well be that the front of your body feels crumpled and collapsed, as though you were trying to curve round your abdomen and protect it. Breathe in, and as you exhale, straighten up and make space in the front of your body – then continue to breathe steadily. You may feel a little tremulous at first, but you will soon feel stronger and braver. This applies at any time when you are feeling closed in around the front of your body because you are upset. By stretching and opening the front of your body you will feel that you literally 'lift your heart'.

Become aware of your feet on the ground and imagine that you are standing in the hard, wet sand at the edge of the sea; visualize your clear, even footprints. Now think of the earth as the mother that can sustain you, even at your most vulnerable. Think of yourself as a plant that can draw up strength through its roots. Imagine your sap rising, up through hips, chest, neck and head, along your arms and into your fingertips. Feel the new energy and potential there, know you are supple and alive. Even if you only experience that aliveness for a fleeting moment, it is enormously helpful to know it can be there.

Standing in *tadasana*, appreciate how brave you are in managing your present loneliness. Withstanding these times makes us very strong and resilient. Connect in your mind with all the other women who have ever been betrayed, abandoned or left in loneliness, and you will begin to get hold of the thread of your own survival.

PARSVAKRONASANA – SIDE FLANK STRETCH
(See page 12)

This strong sideways stretch opens your chest and hips in a powerful extension, and emphasizes strength in the thighs and calves. It helps to stop your chest and abdomen from feeling weak and caved in (as in the benefits of *tadasana* described above), and fills the lower body with life and resilience. Practise equally to each side. The increase in circulation and depth of breathing will help any feelings of numbness and alienation to disappear, and you will feel more fully present in each cell of your body.

ARDHA VIRASANA PASCHIMOTTANASANA – FORWARD STRETCH IN HALF HERO POSE

- Sit in *dandasana*.
- Tuck your right heel around alongside your right buttock.
- Stretch your left heel away, toes pointing to the ceiling.
- Breathe in, sit up tall, stretch your arms up.
- Exhaling, stretch forwards over the straight leg.
- At your comfortable maximum, hold onto the leg, relax your head and neck. Breathe steadily and keep your face and throat relaxed.
- When you want to come up, inhale and lift your head, exhale, release your grip and sit up. Relax your shoulders.
- Repeat the posture, equally attentively, on the other side.

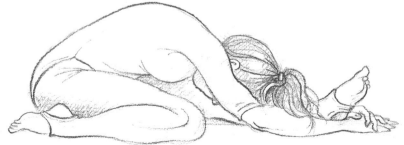

Ardha virasana paschimottanasana (forward stretch in half hero pose)

As well as giving a good stretch to your hips and legs, this posture squeezes and massages your abdomen. It helps to revitalize the area of your body where you may be feeling a lot of your emotional pain.

IN A LOVING PARTNERSHIP

In the first glow of a loving partnership you may feel radiant and tingling, full of physical well-being. You will find more energy and dynamism in your stretches and have a sense of being really alive all over. As the months and years pass, the first outer glow subsides but a steady inner fire may take its place.

The following postures celebrate the warmth and fulfilment of a loving partnership. They should be integrated into the balanced programme you develop for yourself.

The first two are enjoyable poses to practise with someone else. If your partner is also a yoga practitioner you may enjoy the whole range of double yoga poses (see Further reading). Even if your partner is not interested in yoga, doing the double posture with friends at class gives you a chance to explore the nuances, the meanings and the fun of bodies working and cooperating together.

DOUBLE *JANU SIRSASANA* – SHOOTING STAR POSE

- Sit side by side with a partner in *dandasana*.
- Both bring the outside foot in to the perineum or onto the inner thigh in half lotus.
- Inhale and turn towards each other.
- Exhale and stretch forwards, sliding your outside hands to clasp each others' feet, and your inside hands, palm to palm raised behind you.
- Remain as long as you are both comfortable, breathing steadily, faces relaxed and throats soft.
- To come out of the posture, inhale and sit up.
- Next, change sides, and do the pose, just as thoughtfully, once again.

Double
janu sirsasana
(shooting star pose)

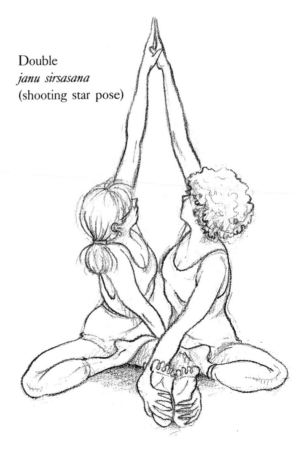

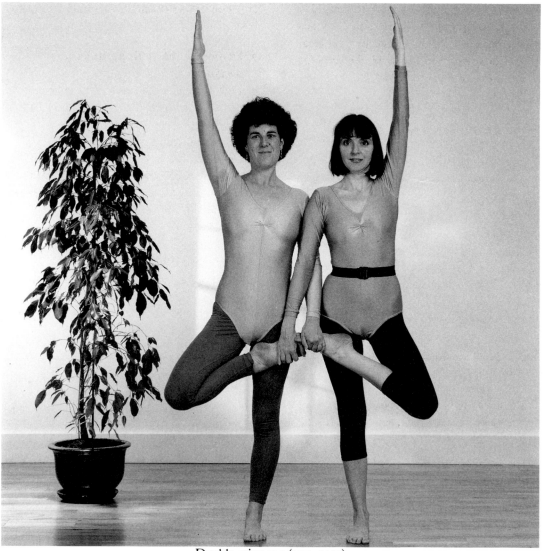

Double *virasana* (tree pose)

DOUBLE *VRKSASANA* – DOUBLE TREE POSE

- Stand with a partner, side by side in *tadasana*.
- Each bring your outer foot up onto the inner thigh.
- Open the bent-knee hip out as far as possible, tuck your tailbone under and lift your abdomen.
- Both focus your gaze on something in front

of you to enhance your balance.
- When you are ready, cross your inside hand in front and hold your partner's foot.
- On an exhalation, each stretch your outside arm up vertically, palm facing in.
- Balance and breathe steadily.
- To come down, float your arms down on an exhalation, and disentangle feet and hands on the next exhalation.
- Next, change sides and do the pose again.

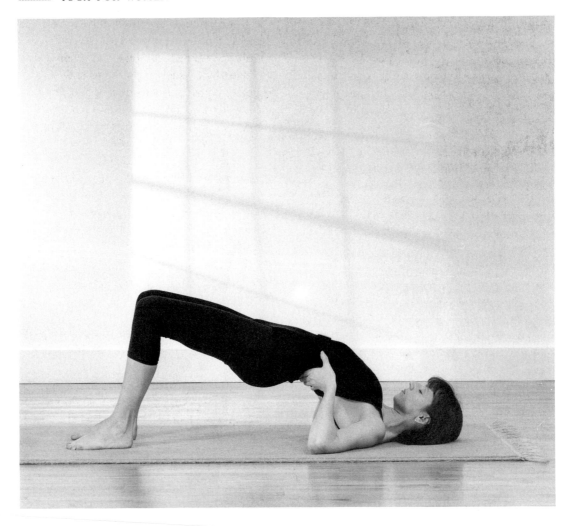

Setu bhandasana (half bridge pose)

SETU BHANDASANA – HALF BRIDGE POSE

This posture has a sensual feel; the upper back is lifted, and the top of the pelvis well stretched out.

- Begin in *salamba sarvangasana*, the shoulder stand.
- Supporting your back with your hands, bring your elbows well in (ideally, your upper arms are parallel on the floor).
- Lift your spine between your shoulder blades and drop your feet to the floor lightly, like a cat.
- Breathe steadily. Make sure your jaw stays soft.
- When you want to come out of the posture, unwind your spine carefully onto the floor.

If your lower back feels tight, hug your knees to your chest and rock slowly from side to side.

VARIATIONS

At first it may be easier to drop one foot first, then the other, to the floor. When you find *setu bhandasana* easy, try walking your feet away from you in the posture until your legs are straight.

OVERSTRESSED

Mental and emotional stress, along with physical stiffness, is one of the invisible epidemics of the last decades of the twentieth century. A certain amount of stress is, of course, challenging and stimulating, and can help us to develop and excel. Beyond a critical point – different for each individual – it becomes destructive. We perform tasks less well, make more errors and begin to suffer from physical manifestations of stress such as disturbances in sleep and digestion, panic attacks accompanied by perhaps palpitations, extra sweating, shallow, fast breathing and so on. We are all familiar with these results of stress, and many of us have experienced some, if not all of them.

Yoga affects stress levels in many ways. Physically speaking, stretching, steady breathing, relaxation and meditation all help to disperse the stress-produced hormones, particularly adrenalin, and encourage the production of hormones which give a sense of well-being.

At a mental or spiritual level, a different perspective on life begins to arise over the weeks and months of practise. This does not imply that one will be any less committed to either career or family, but that there will be less sense of helpless entanglement. A growing sense of the value of inner experience, other people's as well as one's own, of the longer perspective of time and the wider issues of the world, tend to decrease day-to-day stress. This is very valuable to women who may find themselves extended by coordinating a career and children, perhaps also supporting and counselling a worried partner and having an increasing sense of responsibility for ageing parents.

If taking a broad view of the planet brings you another kind of stress, trying to work out what you can do to help preserve the ecosystem, look at Joanna Macey's book, *Despair and Personal Power in the Nuclear Age* (see Further Reading), which helps to find a way of living with the knowledge we have about pollution and arms.

When practising postures, *savasana*, breathing and meditation, the work involves being fully present in the present moment. This continual full attention to each successive second gives a relief from stress and a vivid experience of your own presence in the world. It is described by Dainin Katigiri thus:

We do not realize it, but mind is always picking up activity right at the moment of activity. When you pick up activity, immediately it is form or experience. But right in the midst of activity, there is no form. All you have to do is just be there. This is oneness.

Oneness is the rhythm of the sameness of ocean and you. At that time it is called 'to swim'.
From Returning to Silence: Zen Practice in Everyday Life, *Dainin Katagiri, Shambhala, 1988*

'Just being there' is the freedom from stress inherent in the deepest yoga, being in our own place in the world as fluently as if we were swimming in the ocean. Take care not to let your yoga become another stressor, by getting anxious and guilty if you have not done 'enough'. Do not say to yourself, 'Ought I to do some yoga now?' but, 'Would I like some quiet time for myself? Would I like to spend some of that time on yoga?' Ask yourself, 'What is right for me for today?' and act on that.

The imagery, as well as the physical aspect, of these postures may appeal to you if you are under a lot of stress. Integrate them into your balanced programme.

GARUDASANA – EAGLE POSE

Garudasana is the pose of the eagle. In it the eagle becomes extended and soaring in the sky, then comes down to settle onto its nest, folded and quiet. Performing the pose helps to remind us of moving from extroversion, pouring out of energy and activity to introspection, gathering in of energy, and arriving at a quiet centre.

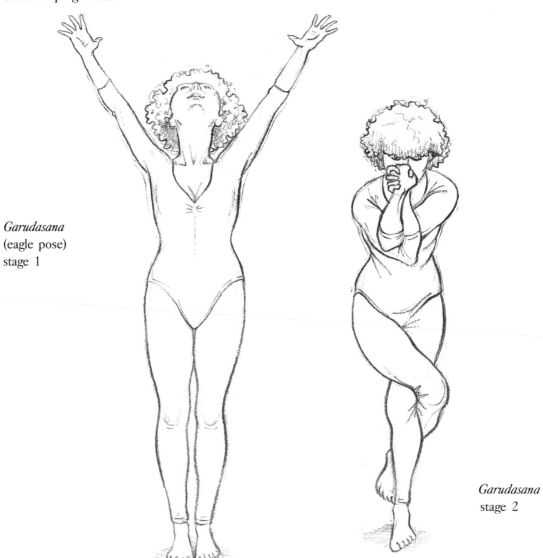

Garudasana
(eagle pose)
stage 1

Garudasana
stage 2

- Inhale and stretch your arms up and wide. Tilt your head back to open your chest and throat.
- Exhale and hook your right leg over left, left arm over right, clasping your hands.
- Bend the standing knee.
- Focus your gaze and balance, breathing steadily.
- To finish the pose, exhale and come into *tadasana*, untangling slowly.
- Now practise *garudasana* on the other side.

SUPTA BADDHA KONASANA – RECLINING COBBLER POSE

It is very relaxing to combine lying down in *savasana* with one of the hip-opening postures, like *baddha konasana* (cobbler pose).

- Sit in *dandasana*.
- Bring the soles of your feet together and flop your knees out to the sides.
- On an exhalation, lean back onto your elbows, then the crown of your head, then slide your shoulders to the floor and lie down, keeping the back of your neck long.
- Place your hands palm to palm together over your heart in *namaste*.
- Think of the back of your waist spreading out. Breathe steadily and rest.
- When you want to finish, straighten your legs, roll over onto your side, and push your hands into the floor to sit up.

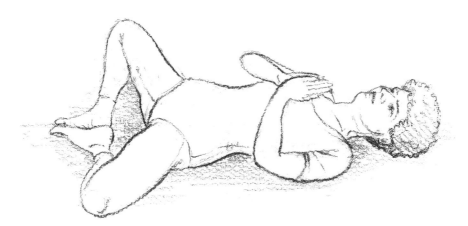

Supta Baddha Konasana
(reclining cobbler pose)

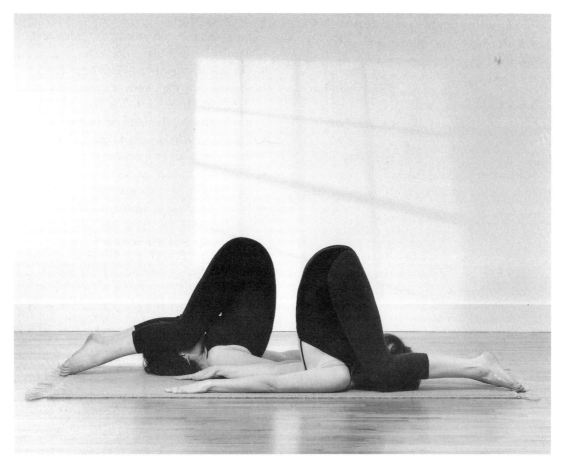

Halasana (plough pose) and *kamapidasana* (knee to ear pose)

HALASANA – PLOUGH POSE
- Start in *salamba sarvangasana*.
- Lift your spine between your shoulder blades and inhale.
- As you exhale, lower your feet lightly to the floor behind your head.
- Keep your jaw relaxed and make as much space as you can between your face and your knees.

- Breathe steadily. If you are quite comfortable, drop your knees down next to your ears in *karnapidasana*.

You will find yourself close to parts of yourself you have not encountered before!

- To come out of *karnapidasana*, return to *halasana* then unwind your spine carefully down onto the floor.

UNDERSTRESSED

It can be as unpleasant to be understressed as it is to be overstressed. As women we are as likely to have parts of our lives when we do not have enough to do, as we are to have stages when we are very hard pressed – for reasons of the fluctuating needs of our families, or of temporary bouts of unemployment due to house moves based on the requirements of partners' careers, or any of the other changes of location or focus that can happen. It is unpleasant to find your skills unused and your talents unchallenged, and not

always easy to know where to begin to find an outlet for their expression.

SURYA NAMASKAR – SALUTE TO THE SUN
The series of postures known as *surya namaskar* or 'salute to the sun' is an enlivening and encouraging exercise.

You will see from the illustration that it includes *tadasana*, the jack-knife (number 3), dog pose (numbers 5 and 8) and cobra pose (number 7) in an invigorating sequence. You can practise in a variety of ways: flowing from one position to the next slowly and remaining

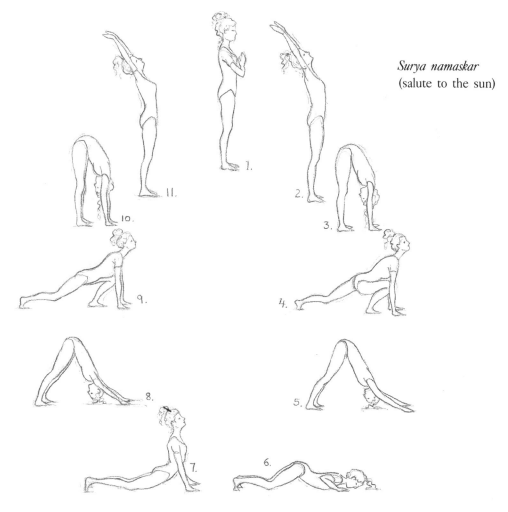

Surya namaskar
(salute to the sun)

for a few seconds in each stretch, or swinging from one position to the next (avoiding any jerkiness or awkwardness) in a faster rhythm without pausing longer in each stage than it takes to extend fully.

Alternate the foot which you step back in position 2 each time you do the sequence. Do a couple of cycles on each side at first. You will find you feel energized and well stretched all over. When you have become more flexible and more fit, you can build up to several cycles on each side.

If you have little time for yoga, a few cycles of *surya namaskar* each day will help to keep you loose, active and in touch with your body.

If you are feeling sluggish, bored and underused, the sequence will help to enliven you, and may help to loosen up your spirit too, enabling you to think of how to enrich your life and become more active and engaged in things which you enjoy and do well.

FEELING FRAGILE

Sometimes it seems to me that the reason women do so much crying is that they do a lot of other people's crying for them as well as their own. Women are often containing the emotions of other family members or friends who are unable to do this for themselves. In addition to this, frequently having to invent and re-invent a structure for an unstructured life, and cope with the physical impact of births, broken nights, crises and emergencies among colleagues, relatives and friends, can leave one feeling brittle and scoured out with strain and emotion.

The postures mentioned in the section on being alone will be helpful here because of their lifting and opening action on the chest and abdomen, and because they strengthen and revive the limbs, helping to stretch any feeling of wilting out of the body. The preliminary breathing exercises described at the end of Chapter 2 are also important. The use of breath to cleanse and refresh in this way can help to counteract the feeling, which is common when in a fragile state, that one can hardly breathe at all because each breath seems to hurt. Think of the breaths flowing into you with a warm and nourishing kindness, and the breaths out taking some of the highly breakable feeling away with them.

VISUALIZATION IN *SAVASANA*

When you feel vulnerable and raw, combine *savasana* with a healing visualization. Read this several times over until it is clear in your mind and you can settle into *savasana* and let it flow in your imagination. You might otherwise prefer to put it onto tape and play it to yourself – if you have a tape-to-tape machine you can put some calm music following on from the visualization to let you continue to enjoy the feeling of peace and wholeness after it has finished. You may have a friend or partner who will read the visualization out to you when you have settled down. If you read onto tape or to a friend, read slowly, with pauses between the phrases as you feel appropriate.

Your body is heavy and relaxed . . . your joints are soft, your muscles warm and relaxed, your shoulders and hips feel heavy and open. Your head is heavy on the floor and your face is soft. Your hands and feet are soft and relaxed. Your spine is releasing more and more. Your breathing is coming and going lightly and steadily in its own rhythm. Your throat is passive and relaxed, and your mind is empty.

You are walking along a path towards a walled garden. There is a gate into the garden, and you are walking towards the gate. Go through the gate into the beautiful garden. The sun is deliciously warm on your body, and you soak up the warmth . . .

In the garden are beautiful flowers and shrubs all around you. Butterflies are dancing in the sunlight. You can smell the lovely scents arising from the warm flowers and you wander among the flower beds enjoying the colours, the shapes, the perfumes . . .

The sun is warm, it is peaceful, quiet and sleepy, just the occasional murmuring of bees or birdsong arises from time to time in the silence . . .

In the middle of the garden is a pool of clear, clean water. You walk to the pool and dip yourself into the clear, clean sparkling water. All your tiredness, sadness and confusion is washed away in the crystal water of the pool.

Come out of the pool fresh and clean, newly born, and lay yourself down to dry in the warm sunshine, surrounded by the beauty of the garden . . .

Allow yourself as much time as you want and need to rest at the end of the visualization. When you are ready to bring your awareness back into the room and the situation you are in, do so by lengthening your breath a little, stretching first your fingers and toes, then your arms and legs, and having a good yawn, before you blink your eyes open and roll over onto your side, pushing your hands into the floor to sit yourself up.

If you enjoyed this guided fantasy, you will find more in Chapter 5.

VERY FIT

In contrast with the days or weeks when our consciousness of ourselves is of a breakable little shell, there are times too when we feel strong, magnificent, sturdy and marvellous. These strong poses are enjoyable to attempt while you are celebrating your strength. However exuberant you feel, do not forget all the usual cautions about not forcing, going in your own time to the rhythm of your own breathing, and not allowing pride or ego to cause you to rush. Having said that, with careful attention you can enjoy the resources of your capable and delightful body. Any time you are able to feel this positive awareness of your own body, or share the feeling with others, or help to awaken this feeling in them, you are helping to free women from the cruel tyranny of physical stereotypes, and reclaim the joy of the physical self, the miraculous organism made of the materials you have borrowed from the universe for the duration of this physical life.

VIRABHADRASANA III – WARRIOR POSE III
The third of the warrior cycle, this powerful balance is tough to do but very enjoyable.

- Start in *virabhadrasana I*.
- As you exhale, bend the front knee and lift the back foot off the floor.
- Straighten the standing leg and stretch the lifted heel away. Extend your chest and arms parallel to the floor.
- Take your gaze to your stretched fingertips.
- Breathe steadily with your face relaxed.
- To come out of the posture, return to *virabhadrasana I*.
- When your breathing and heartbeat have returned to normal, turn and practise *virabhadrasana III* to the other side.

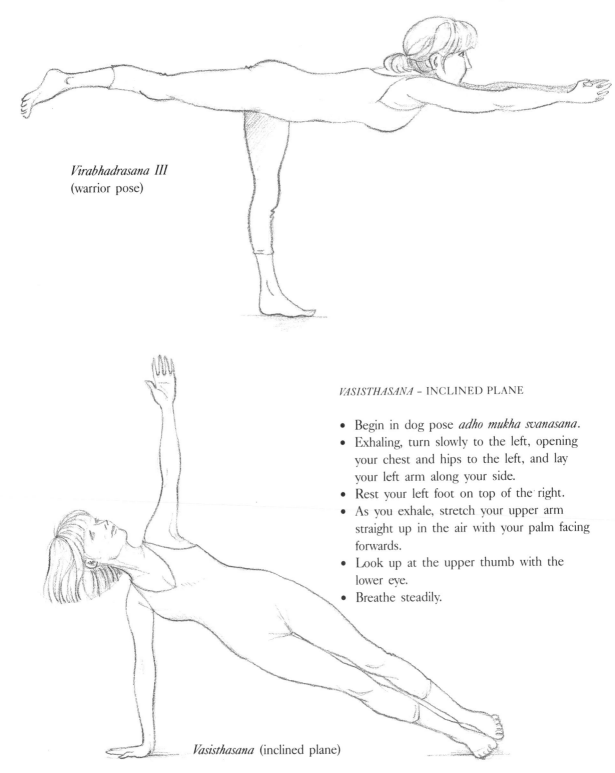

Virabhadrasana III
(warrior pose)

VASISTHASANA – INCLINED PLANE

- Begin in dog pose *adho mukha svanasana*.
- Exhaling, turn slowly to the left, opening your chest and hips to the left, and lay your left arm along your side.
- Rest your left foot on top of the right.
- As you exhale, stretch your upper arm straight up in the air with your palm facing forwards.
- Look up at the upper thumb with the lower eye.
- Breathe steadily.

Vasisthasana (inclined plane)

- To come out of the posture, return to dog pose, then sit back in the praying stretch.
- When your breathing and heartbeat have returned to normal, do *vasisthasana* to the other side.

NATARAJASANA – LORD OF THE DANCE

Nataraja is one of the names for *Siva*, the Cosmic Dancer. The pose is beautiful, but harder than it looks, requiring great flexibility in hips, back and shoulders.

- Stand in *tadasana*.
- Focus your gaze to enhance your balance.
- Bend your left knee and draw it up behind you with your left hand.
- When the foot is at your comfortable maximum, reach behind you with your right hand and catch the foot with this hand too.
- Breathe steadily, and think of bringing lightness and life to your whole body.

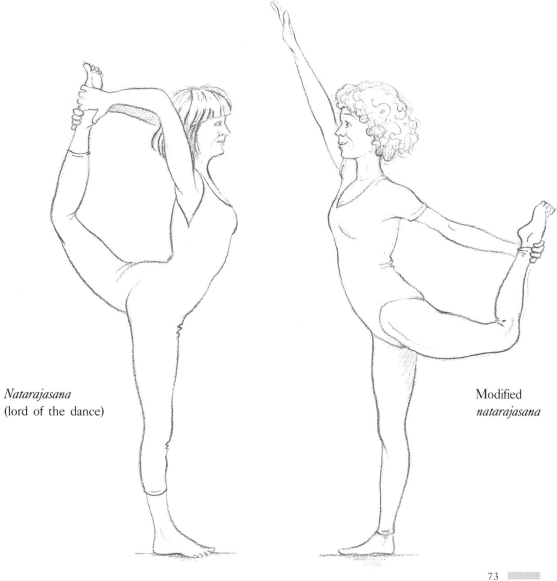

Natarajasana
(lord of the dance)

Modified
natarajasana

- To come out of the pose, release the foot and lower hands and foot slowly and with control.
- Practise *natarajasana* on the other foot.

VARIATION

At first it is useful to hold the foot with the same-side hand and stretch the other arm up.

This allows the body to become flexible gradually.

Some adepts are able to rest the head back onto the instep of the lifted foot! Never force the pace of this powerful stretch. The circle is the cycle of creation and destruction – the dance of life.

CHAPTER FIVE

IMAGE AND LIFESTYLE

Physical asanas are the route through which the majority of us in the West find our way to yoga. These asanas, however, are only part of yoga, so in this chapter we look at the guidance and interpretations we may find in yoga for a variety of different aspects of our lives.

EATING, SIZE AND WEIGHT

Moderate diet means pleasant, sweet food, leaving free one fourth of the stomach.
Hatha Yoga Pradipika, *1:58*

Let's take the quality of the food and the quantity of the food as two separate issues. What, from the yoga point of view, is 'pleasant, sweet food'? Food, as well as all the other substances in the physical world, intangibles such as actions and motives, are divided into three different basic qualities known as the *gunas*: *sattva* (representing purity), *rajas* (representing activity, passion and the process of change) and *tamas* (representing darkness and inertia). These three qualities exist in the universe in a constantly shifting equilibrium, and are only transcended in a state of enlightenment.

The *sattvic* foods include cereals, wholemeal bread, fresh fruit, fresh vegetables, pure fruit juices, milk, butter, cheese, legumes, nuts, seeds and honey.

Rajasic foods include anything that is very hot, bitter, sour, dry or salty. Sharp spices and strong herbs are *rajasic*, as are coffee and tea, fish, eggs, salt and chocolate. It is considered *rajasic* to eat food in a hurry.

Tamasic foods include meat, alcohol, tobacco, onions, garlic, fermented foods, vinegar, and also anything which is stale or overripe. Overeating is *tamasic*.

The 'pleasant, sweet food' of the *Pradipika* refers to foods in the *sattvic* category, and we can aim gradually to eat more and more foods in the *sattvic* group, and less and less foods from the *rajasic* and *tamasic* types. Apply to any changes in your eating pattern the same attitude as you apply to your postures and your preliminary breathing exercises: that is, don't force anything, don't do anything that feels violent or awkward or extreme. Find that point of equilibrium in action where you are making choices not out of guilt, loyalty or dogma, but because those choices have arisen genuinely inside you. Eat a wide variety of foods within the *sattvic* category and, if you find you want less meat as you practise yoga more, be sure to have plenty of protein from other sources (nuts, pulses, cheese and milk).

Sattvic foods may look very bland at first and you may be alarmed at the thought of 'giving up' hot spices or coffee, for example. However, it is probably better not to see it as an exercise in cutting things out of your intake, but rather noticing and allowing yourself to follow an increasing desire for fresh, rather plain food, and then enjoying the light, clean feeling that evolves from that.

Our planet is so polluted that it is very difficult to find foods free of excessive chemical toxins. It is, by now, probably impossible to find any food completely free of such substances which are spread throughout the soil, the air, the rain and the oceans worldwide. We have to accept the fact that we can no longer clean up our food and our insides by taking individual responsibility for doing so, and understand with sorrow that it is already too late for that. What we can do is to wash all fresh fruits and vegetables thoroughly to rid them as much as possible of pesticides and lead, and use organically grown vegetables and grains where possible. We can be aware that both the antibiotics and the growth hormones fed to farm animals are present in most of the meat in the shops, and look out for organically raised meat if we want to eat meat. Fish absorb the waste poisons dissolved in the sea and rivers – the deeper swimming fish tend to be the cleanest, and fish such as eels and mussels which live in the shallows, the most polluted.

We can do our best to sort out our own food and eating, and to be informed and aware of news and research about pollution and its effects on ourselves and our families via the food we eat. The anger and sadness that we feel about this may prompt us to look for social as well as personal changes. In this everyone has to make her own choices about her own actions and her own boundaries.

The quantity of food to be eaten is clearly described: '. . . leaving free one fourth of the stomach.' Most animals eat what they need and no more. Half the human population of planet earth cannot find enough to eat at the end of the twentieth century. Those of us in the fraction living in the affluent West often overeat. We have a very complicated relationship with quantity of food which leaves us in difficulty recognizing what it would feel like 'leaving free one fourth of the stomach', and even if we could sense what that was, we might find it difficult to stop eating there.

The rules, punishments and rewards concerning food which we experienced when we were children may have an effect on how we feel in our adult lives about the amount we eat. Women who were children in the UK when food was still rationed in the 1940s and early 1950s may have been aware of the adults' anxiety about food, whether there would be enough, and may have been very clearly instructed to eat everything they were given whether they felt hungry or not. Any woman who grew up with these pressures may feel obliged to 'eat up' leftovers, and always to finish everything on the plate. She may still carry a fear that there may not be enough food to last, so that nothing must ever be wasted, whether her body needs anything at that particular time or not. Although no-one would advocate wasting food, it may be useful to work on realizing that there is a choice, that food does not have to be finished up compulsively when it is not appropriate.

Women a decade or more younger may have been children when sweets finally came off ration in the early 1950s. Parents were delighted to be able to provide their children with sweets at last, and many of us had sweets every day for years through our childhood and, furthermore, the sweets were associated with rewards and pleasure, and withholding sweets was a form of punishment. Many of us thus connected having refined sugars as a way of being nice to ourselves and other people, and came to associate a lack of sweets and chocolates with bleakness and punishment. Again, we may wish to re-examine that relationship with sweets so that we can choose when and how much to have of them with fewer of the emotional complications.

Still younger women may have had their relationship with food affected by the growth of the fast food industry, and become accustomed to large amounts of highly processed foods of all kinds. Social restrictions on having snacks between meals and on eating while moving around were relaxed and many people have become used to eating something as soon as they feel even a little bit hungry, rather than eating regular meals in-between which they expected to feel hungry at times. A change to more fresh wholefoods should be made gradually in order to let the digestive system accustom itself to fresh foodstuffs. Equally, a change to regular meals with spaces in-between rather than a continual stream of snacks should be negotiated gradually.

In spite of the fact that women in the Third World spend their entire lives trying to find enough to eat, many of us in the West are pulled into the cultural obsession to be thin, and disrupt our eating patterns and our metabolisms by repeatedly going on and off more or less radical diets. The desperation to control our weight and size can sometimes become a metaphor for an attempt to control our lives and identities, and when that happens the acute suffering of anorexia nervosa and bulimia nervosa may become a possibility.

If you feel larger than is comfortable for you, you might want to consider gradually eating smaller quantities of fat, and moderate quantities of complex carbohydrates, filling up more with vegetables and fruits. Towards the end of a meal, think about leaving a fourth of your stomach free. Don't tense up about it, but think about how full or not you feel. Give yourself a few moments to make a choice about whether to go on eating or not. Notice the difference between how your abdomen feels when you have filled your stomach up completely, and when you leave it a little empty. Do what feels right for you at that particular moment, and also notice how you feel in the following few hours and whether your decision has affected that or not. We can gradually learn to eat only what we need, but it takes time and we need to be patient with ourselves.

Kim Chernin's book, *The Hungry Self* (see Further Reading) looks at women's struggles with a bulimic relationship with food and identity, and Sheila Macleod's *The Art of Starvation* (see Further Reading) tells her own story of episodes of anorexia. These books are useful to all women because they illuminate the way in which food and identity have become tangled for women. If you or anybody close to you is suffering from anorexia or bulimia, you must understand that these are life-threatening conditions and seek help through your GP or by going straight to a centre specializing in eating disorders. Practising yoga is an excellent way to help to rebuild a loving relationship with the physical self, and to dismantle punitive and destructive feelings about the body, and is therefore useful to any woman suffering in this way.

To sum up, then, gradual change to a moderate, *sattvic* diet without making a fetish of it and learning to eat to about three-quarters fullness and to stop there, again without making a battle of will and self-discipline about it, should help to make our bodies arrive at the size and weight that is comfortable, healthy and appropriate for us as individuals.

Consider the *gunas* once again: *sattva* meaning purity, *rajas* meaning activity and passion and *tamas* meaning inertia and darkness. Once you have absorbed the idea of these categories you can see how they could apply to other substances, and also attitudes and forms of behaviour: for instance, you can imagine the differences between *rajasic* touch, *tamasic* touch and *sattvic* touch, differences which would be important in massage or even the most informal kind of healing touch. Consider making *sattvic* choices a greater part of your life in order to increase your feeling of well-being and inner quiet. It may seem unlikely that you could prioritize *sattvic* behaviour in, say, a business context or on a social occasion, but it does not actually involve being weak, passive or dull, rather a peaceful alertness and a liveliness that comes from inner aliveness instead of a brittle performance. Do not allow these considerations to make you become self-conscious and confused – simply carry the idea around with you and see how and where it might apply usefully for you.

CHAKRA, COLOUR AND SOUND

The *chakras* are energy centres which lie along the centre line of the body. Each *chakra* relates to particular activities, moods and qualities, as well as colours and sounds.

Some practitioners of yoga regard the existence of the *chakras* as the literal truth, some would see them as symbolic or metaphorical. It is a matter for each person to

work out for herself, and indeed one's views may change as one makes a stronger link with yoga. The location of the *chakras* corresponds with plexuses in the physical body, but this does not either prove or disprove that they 'really' exist.

We may also notice that there is a congruence between some of our own cultural locations for feelings in the body, such as putting our hand over our heart, which corresponds to *anahata chakra*, the *chakra* for emotional harmony, while describing strong emotions; or pressing the fingers into *ajna chakra*, between the eyebrows, which is the *chakra* for intellectual activity, when we are struggling to understand a complicated concept. This does not 'prove' or 'disprove' the existence of the *chakras* either, but it is an interesting resonance.

Perhaps the most useful approach is to begin by assuming that the *chakras* are an interesting set of symbols – like, for example, Jung's archetypes of the collective unconscious – and see what insight and growth proceeds from responding to them at that level. You can then see whether a further sense of the meaning of the *chakras* develops for you later on.

Colours in the Chakras
Each *chakra* has a corresponding colour. When you imagine the location of the *chakra*, imagine a glow of its colour in that place. You may also like to think of the colours which you enjoy wearing in terms of their *chakra* meaning, and sometimes to choose clothes, or even a small item such as a scarf or jewellery, of a colour to vibrate with the *chakra* energy you feel you need. We are all aware of the fact that our sense of confidence and well-being is influenced by the clothes we wear, and that something that 'feels' right and looks

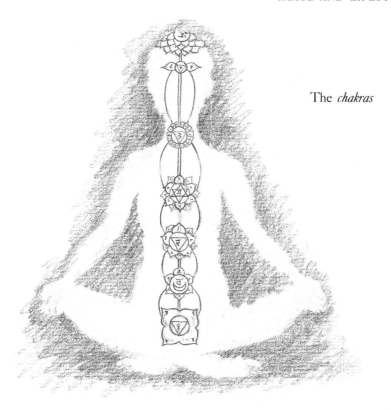

The *chakras*

lovely one day may feel and look quite incongruous the next.

Muladhara chakra is situated at the perineum. Its colour is red, and wearing red or red objects helps to stabilize and earth a person. There are many different reds – look carefully – some sing with an undertone of yellow and orange, some with vibrations of blue and violet. Some are a pure tulip red. If your red has undertones of other colours, it will carry a slight undercurrent of those *chakra* energies too.

The activities associated with *muladhara chakra* are action, sensation and reproduction, and the mental process is that of establishing facts.

Swadisthana chakra is located at the prostatic plexus and relates to the colour orange. Orange is a propitious colour for interaction and making changes, and helps with sociability. You may like to wear orange clothes or accessories if interaction with others is important for you at a particular time.

Activities associated with *swadisthana chakra* are social interaction; the mental process is that of relating and making comparisons.

Manipura chakra sits at the solar plexus and its colour is yellow. Wearing yellow helps to support the ego and self-confidence, and is an antidote to depression. Think of how your heart lifts when you see the first daffodils of spring! The colour is a wonderful celebration.

Pale-skinned northern races hesitate to wear yellow, since the colour seems to drain tone from a white skin, but if you are white-skinned, look for a yellow with a golden undertone rather than with a blue or a lime undertone, and you will find it easy enough to wear.

Activities which relate to the *manipura chakra* are intellectual explanations and analysis.

Moving up the *sushumna*, the central channel of energy corresponding to the spinal cord in the physical body, the next *chakra* is *anahata* at roughly heart level. Its function is to harmonize at the emotional level, and its colour is green. Green is a pleasant colour to wear if you feel crowded, rushed or pressurized emotionally, but should be avoided if you are feeling over-emotional, as it will only activate your emotions even more. Be aware of the undertone colours in any green you choose.

Anahata-based activities are the search for security and self-esteem.

Vissudha chakra is in the throat and its colour is blue. The *vissudha* activities are study, learning, absorbing facts – not so much the intellectual-insight side of study which is the province of *ajna*, but more the hard work and application, highly verbal and logical side of study and learning. Perhaps scholastic organizations are inclined also to have particular songs linked with them to refresh *vissudha chakra* with singing after long hours of study! Blue is a good colour to aid concentration, receptivity, and learning.

The activities linked with *vissudha* are being in authority, learning about the past, and synthesizing data into concepts.

Ajna chakra sits in the third eye position between and slightly above the eyebrows. It is linked, as already mentioned, with intellectual insights, and with intuition and psychic qualities. Its colour is indigo.

The activities linked with it are direct perception and intuition.

Sahasraha chakra is the thousand-petalled lotus at the crown of the head. It radiates a pure and spiritual quality. The location of *sahasraha chakra* is the same as is highlighted by haloes in the religious paintings of Western art. The colours linked with *sahasraha* are white and violet. Many cultures use white garments to signify purity, especially on ceremonial occasions. White silk often has a delightful violet tinge, combining the two colours together.

The activities which arise from *sahasraha* are envisioning and the creation of images.

It would probably be a mistake to begin putting on clothes as it were 'for luck', linked with the *chakra* colours, in an artificial manner. It would leave you feeling self-conscious and silly. You might find it interesting, though, to think about the different colours you have chosen to wear in different parts of your life and notice whether they link in with the *chakras* in any way. I notice, for example, that when I first began yoga, long before I had heard anything about the *chakras*, I bought a red leotard. When this disintegrated a couple of years later I chose a green one, and on its demise a blue one was selected, still not having any idea what the colours might 'mean' in the *chakric* sense. Most of my life I have worn predominantly blue clothes and am indeed inclined to be rather bookish and very verbal.

In terms of choosing clothes, be intuitive about what you want to wear, rather than trying deliberately to pick the 'right' colour for the situation you anticipate. If you choose intuitively, you will often see in retrospect that you picked exactly the colour you needed.

The shape and texture of clothes can be thought of in terms of the *gunas*. As we discussed with relation to food, you will probably find that a desire to wear *sattvic* shapes and textures (natural fibres, fluid, highly physical, unrestrictive shapes) will evolve as you become more and more involved with your yoga practice. There is no need at all to begin changing artificially, as an affectation. It happens by itself in time.

Sound and the Chakras

The energy of colour affects us in one way and the energy of sound affects us in another way. All of us have experienced both the location of different kinds of sounds from our own voices within our own bodies and also the profound effect on our emotional and spiritual state of hearing different sounds.

Think of how your voice rings in your own ears and vibrates in the skull area if you shriek or squeal. When you hum gently you may feel a warm buzzing feeling in the lips and a pleasant vibration in the rib cage. If you have experienced childbirth, you may recall extraordinary noises coming out of you quite involuntarily while you pushed the baby out – deep groaning sounds having a definitely pelvic origin. Sound can certainly be experienced in all sorts of ways and qualities throughout the body.

As for the emotional aspect, strong feelings can clearly be released by sound. Most of us find rhythmic sounds, the waves breaking on the beach, breezes rustling in the trees, very soothing. A sudden noise on a silent night can send a shudder up the spine. If a breeze grows to a hurricane, the sound of nature becoming violent makes the skin prickle, and the hair at the nape of the neck stirs, while the pulse races. Gentle crooning or singing are soothing to hear from the earliest age, and if the song or tune is one we know, strong associative processes will bring back old emotions, sometimes very poignantly.

The sounds used in the yoga discipline are known as *mantram* (*man*: thinking; *tra*: a means of). Each *chakra* has its own *mantra*. While you repeat it you focus your awareness on the *chakra*.

When there is an 'a' sound in the middle of the *mantra* it is pronounced as a long 'ah'. The 'o' sound in the last two *mantram* is a long 'oh'. The *mantram* are as follows:

muladhara chakra	LAM
swadisthana chakra	VAM
manipura chakra	RAM
anahata chakra	YAM
vissudha chakra	HAM
ajna chakra	OM (shorter)
sahasraha chakra	OM (longer)

If you want to try chanting, begin by sitting with the spine lifting upright from its root to the skull and with your chest lifting and open, your shoulders releasing back and down. Relax your hips and knees in a cross-legged position or, if you are comfortable in either *siddhasana* or *padmasana* (the lotus pose), either of those would be suitable. Take your time getting established in a poised position, lifting but relaxed.

Let your eyes close and let your breathing steady itself into a rhythm. When your breathing is steady, inhale, pause momentarily, then begin to chant. If you are chanting a *mantra* with three sounds in it, use about a third of the breath on each sound, and let the breath flow out at a steady pace. Choose any note you like, and experience the sound vibrating in your body. If you are using one of the *chakra mantram*, take your awareness to the site of the appropriate *chakra*.

When the breath is finished and the sound has died away, inhale at an even rate, without strain, and chant again. You will probably find five or six repetitions of the *mantra* will be enough at first.

It is refreshing to start at *muladhara chakra*, and chant the *mantra* for each *chakra* in turn, repeating each the same number of times, moving up the *sushumna*.

When you come to *ajna chakra*, the 'om' is chanted on a relatively high note and repeated several times with each breath rather like a bell chiming. *Sahasraha chakra* has a long 'om', where you think of the sound originating deep down in the hips and gradually flowing upwards to the crown of the head. It may be useful to feel the 'om' sound made of the flowing together of the sounds 'Ah-Oh-Mm'.

Approach chanting without strain or self-consciousness. The initial sense of oddness will soon fade. If you ever become dizzy, stop at once and let your breathing come to an everyday level until you are comfortable again. When you chant again, do not 'try' quite so hard. Think of pacing the breath out, with its sound, gently and evenly.

When you become used to chanting, its initial effect is that mixture of soothing and energizing which is so characteristic of yoga practices. Later the repetition of *mantra* leads

to a meditative state, stilling the current of thought and opening the door to an experience of oneness.

When you have become used to repeating a *mantra* out loud, you will find that it is also possible to concentrate on silent repetitions of the mantra and arrive at a similar state of peace and stillness.

YAMA AND *NIYAMA* – ON NOT GOING TO EXTREMES

Yoga gives guidelines on what might be called attitude or lifestyle. The *yamas* and *niyamas* are moral precepts which are prerequisites to the practice of yoga – in the eight-fold path (see Chapter 1) they come *before* posture (*asana*) and breathing/*prana* disciplines (*pranayama*). The frame of mind in which you undertake all your practice should be based on the *yamas* and *niyamas*. What precisely each *yama* and *niyama* means, and what its applications and limits are in your own life, is a matter for each person to work out, and frequently review in the light of experience.

Yama

The *yamas* are listed briefly on the following pages.

AHIMSA – NON-VIOLENCE

The concept of *ahimsa* needs careful thought. Does it for you include violence to humans? to animals? to the planet? Would offending somebody else's ideals count as violence for you? What if the other person was behaving in a way that you regard as over-sensitive? Where does your responsibility end and theirs begin? Would encroaching on the spirit of an occasion be violent in your view? These distinctions can only be arrived at with careful thought.

SATYA – TRUTHFULNESS

Clearly we all aim to be truthful over really important issues. However, is it all right to lie in order to oil the social wheels from time to time? Is it acceptable to lie to protect someone else? Is the literal truth more important than being true to the ideals of kindness and friendliness? Are there times when it is important to speak the truth even though it might hurt somebody else?

ASTEYA – NON-STEALING

Few of us steal other people's property. Is it equally important not to steal their time, or their credit, or their opportunities?

BRAHMACHARYA – CELIBACY

What does celibacy mean for us in our culture? Does it mean abstaining from sex altogether? Or does it mean abstaining from compulsive and exploitative sex? Perhaps the latter is more applicable, perhaps it is to do with looking at how you choose to spend your potential energy, and how you deal with very vivid sensations and experiences. Perhaps the concept of *brahmacharya* extends to other experiences where you might get drawn into a compulsive or exploitative reaction – the use of drugs or alcohol for example; or perhaps it applies to relationships other than sexual ones where the issues of possessiveness, faithfulness and integrity could still arise.

Historically, some gurus have been literally celibate, while others have had partners and families. In paintings and drawings you will see some teachers sitting on tiger skins, and some on antelope skins. Only a complete celibate is permitted to sit on a tiger skin.

In the Eastern literature about yoga there is little reference to celibacy with regard to women. It is, however, a powerful theme in medieval Christian culture that a woman could increase her power, energy, and possible range of action in the world by becoming a member of a celibate order. She could also enter a contemplative celibate order and become an extremely powerful person and symbol in spiritual terms, and could claim special social status, respect, and rights as a result of her celibate state.

In the late nineteenth and early twentieth centuries women had to make a clear choice between marriage and entry into professions such as teaching or the civil service. This is not to say that they were necessarily celibate if unmarried, but probably some of them were. The restriction on employment seems to suggest the residual feeling that a woman's finite amounts of potential energy had to be spent in properly chosen channels – either a family or a career but not both. Few of us would wish to return to any such restrictive practices and, indeed, seek instead to improve the balance between family and career by suggesting that male partners direct more energy into the home situation rather than women less into their careers. However, few women find the integration of multiple roles simple. It may be what we want and have a right to, but it isn't easy.

Until the second half of the twentieth century celibacy was the only sure way for a woman to know that her work, efforts and development would not be punctuated by a regular stream of pregnancies, miscarriages and births.

Speaking in 1989, 18 years after the publication of *The Female Eunuch*, Germaine Greer reflected that, at present, women seemed to be liberated, only to be permanently exhausted; that they had successfully fought for the right for key jobs in the professions but had continued to do all their other types of work as well.

With these things in mind, the precept of *brahmacharya* may give a woman, as well as an opportunity to reflect on strategies and philosophies for avoiding compulsive and exploitative sex and sexuality, a chance to think carefully about the distribution of her energies generally, and whether they are being used in the ways which she would positively choose.

APARIGRAHA – NON-COVETOUSNESS

Aparigraha refers to not coveting objects belonging to someone else, as in the familiar Biblical commandment.

We need to consider whether it has any further meanings for us. Does it, for instance, extend to not coveting another person's talents and abilities, or physique, or career, or opportunities? Maybe it does.

Aparigraha further implies non-attachment to anything. Nothing, in the last analysis, really belongs to anybody. The body I live in, composed of and functioning by its use of gases, plants and animals that I consume and transform, can hardly be said to belong to me. It seems much more like something that I borrow, do my best or worst with, but ultimately have to give back to the universe after a number of years. Any abilities I have certainly do not belong to me – they evolve out of my circumstances and the way I choose to respond to those circumstances, but they can hardly be said to be property of mine.

Women have, very appropriately through the feminist movement, made efforts to reclaim

their bodies from male definition, to name and celebrate their skills, strengths and abilities. I have participated in this growth and been much strengthened and empowered by it – and practice of *aparigraha* need not undermine anybody's self-esteem – but it can suggest a perspective for assessing who owns what in the universe which may be useful.

As with the postures, the breathing, the rest of yoga, consider the *yamas* in whatever way and to whatever extent is useful for you for today. There is no need to come to definitive conclusions. They are like a crystal you might look at and see different refractions on different occasions – all of them real.

Niyama

Niyamas are not so much about the interactions between people as about one's frame of mind and way of living. It may be useful to reflect on these.

SAUCHA – PURITY

Saucha includes outer cleanliness like bathing and cleaning the body, and inner cleanliness affected by the practice of *pranayama*, and by *sattvic* eating.

Saucha also refers to a purity of the mind and spirit. Women have suffered so much from being the 'angel in the house', from being expected in this culture to be the 'nice' ones in any situation: pacific, diplomatic, flexible and generous, that this precept of mental *saucha* may be hard to contemplate. It does not, in my view, involve being passive, weak, or exploited. It implies rather a commitment and development towards positive and clear thought and action. It may militate against harbouring grudges, but it does not mean you have to give up righteous anger either on behalf of yourself as an individual, of women as a group, or of causes or issues about which you feel strongly. You do have an obligation to develop your thinking as lucidly as possible in order to make as clear a distinction as you can between unnecessary negative feelings and just anger, and to act positively to make such changes as you can when you feel your anger is just.

This is a personal interpretation of mine, showing clearly my reaction to an upbringing which conditioned me to be 'nice', hence my feeling of being very threatened by any instruction which seems to repeat that pressure to repress 'not nice' feelings or states of mind. No doubt some women will share that kind of conditioning and therefore arrive at a similar interpretation to mine. Others will have grown up in different contexts with different pressures and have different views. The important thing is to work out what the concept means for you in your particular life.

SANTOSA – CONTENTMENT

Santosa is contentment or tranquillity. Again, it does not mean helpless passivity, or pretending to like things which you do not like. It means, perhaps, a kind of acknowledgement of the reality of each minute as it comes along, such as is often described by the Zen teachers. A man who had a very tedious and demanding job asked Taknan, a Zen teacher, to suggest how he could get through the time. Taknan wrote eight Chinese characters and gave them to the man:

> Not twice this day
> Inch foot time gem

The interpretation is, 'This day will not come again. Each moment is a priceless gem.' (*Zen Flesh, Zen Bones*, Anecdote 32, see Further Reading).

I feel this does not mean that every day is lovely if only you look at it properly, but that every day is unique, and your unique self interacting with this unique day has its own unrepeatable and valuable flavour, whatever that may be. Reflection on this helps to dispel the discontent that arises when our days pass in a sort of grey soup, and a strange contentment, even in the presence of pain, pressure and other negative experiences can arise. At times it grows to a vivid pleasure about being in the world at all, whatever the conditions of one's life:

> *There is nothing to see through our six senses. But when we sit down, we can exactly encounter what-is-just-is. Also within what-is-just-is, which is called buddha, we can become one with winter, trees, birds, all sentient beings, exactly.*
> Returning to Silence, *Dainin Katigiri, p. 55*

Perhaps that feeling of belonging in, and identification with, the world, is where contentment can begin – or perhaps that is only where it begins for me. Ask yourself where it may begin for you.

TAPAS – AUSTERITY

Tapas comes from the root word 'tap' which means to burn, or blaze, or be radiant or brilliant. It may be thought of as the burning heat of effort and enthusiasm, or as a purifying fire which burns away the clutter of old anxieties, confusions and repressed emotions.

Most of us have an aspect which burns brightly – *tapas* acknowledges and celebrates this. It challenges us to consider whether we are burning in the place and in the way that we really would choose to burn: that is, are our best efforts and enthusiasms being used where we feel they really are best used.

SVADHYAYA – STUDY

Sva means 'self', and *adhyaya* means study or education, so *svadhyaya* means 'education of the self' or 'study conducive to knowledge of the self'. Any activity which leads to exploration or enrichment of the self is practice of *svadhyaya*.

ISHVARAPRANIDHANA – SURRENDER TO *ISHVARA*

Ishvara means the subtlest level of creation – the essence of creativity. *Ishvarapranidhana* means the dedication of all actions and thoughts, hopes and aspirations, to creativity, to growth and development, to positivity, energy and love. It implies a detachment from the short-term results and rewards for actions, and a commitment to act for the best without attachment.

YOGA NIDRA

Yoga Nidra is a form of meditation where the body is sleeping but the mind is awake. The aim is to experience a deep restfulness while at the same time being completely alert.

Lie down and arrange yourself on the floor in *savasana*, corpse pose. Make sure your centre line is straight, your shoulders and hips open and soft, and the back of your neck long. Feel how your head is heavy on the floor and your body is soft and heavy, your limbs relaxed and your toes and fingers soft.

First of all, observe your breathing. Do not interfere with the breathing at all, just observe it. Do not sleep. Your body is becoming softer, heavier, more relaxed, but your mind is calm and alert.

When your breath has settled into its own natural rhythm, begin to count your breaths. The breath in is one, the breath out is two, and so on. Count up to seven and then go back to the beginning, and count to seven again. Continue with this for a few minutes. Do not fall asleep. Observe gently as you become more deeply relaxed.

Now take your awareness to each part of the body in turn. Just observe the body, do not sleep. Begin with the toes on your left foot. Be aware of each toe in turn, then the foot, the ball of the foot, the top of the foot, the heel. Take your awareness to your calf, your knee, your thigh, your hip. Do not sleep.

Go to the right foot and be aware of each toe in turn. Think of the ball of the right foot, the top of the foot, the heel. Be aware of the calf, the knee, the thigh, the hip. Pause and observe each part. Take your time – but do not sleep.

Become aware of your abdomen, the left side of your waist, the right side of your waist, then the left side of your chest, the right side of your chest.

Take your awareness to your left shoulder, upper arm, elbow, forearm, and wrist. Be aware of your left palm, of each finger, and your thumb. Do the same on the right side – shoulder, upper arm, elbow, forearm, wrist, palm, and fingers and thumb.

Think of your neck and throat, your face, your head.

Now think of your whole body. Do not sleep. Let the time pass, floating by.

When you want to surface again, breathe a little more deeply, yawn and stretch. Open your eyes and become used to the light.

Stretch and wriggle until you feel ready to roll over onto your side, and push your hands into the floor to sit yourself up.

Sometimes people experience the observing action of yoga nidra as a light or glow of warmth travelling around the body. Sometimes it seems like a lightly stroking hand. This form of relaxation is simple but very effective. Practised once or twice a week it will link you into a lake of calmness and strength which will be a great resource for you.

You may like to read and re-read the instructions until you are familiar with them, or ask a friend to read the instructions out slowly to you, with plenty of pauses, or put the instructions onto a tape. If you tape yoga nidra, you might like to add some peaceful music on the end, to accompany your complete relaxation, or you may just prefer to be in the silence.

VISUALIZATION

This guided fantasy can be used in a similar way to the one described in Chapter 4. Either familiarize yourself with it and then settle down and follow the visualization through for yourself, taking your time and allowing yourself to notice what arises for you, or ask a friend to read through the visualization, leaving plenty of long pauses. Another possibility is to make a tape of the visualization, perhaps adding some gentle music after the final words so that you can continue to lie and enjoy the peace.

Clear a space on the floor and switch off the telephone. Lie yourself down comfortably, with the centre line of your body straight, roll your legs and arms outwards until you have a feeling of your shoulders and hips being open.

If you want to, shift your shoulder blades down a little towards your hips. Sometimes it is useful to be aware of what your 'leading' shoulder is doing (right side if you are right-handed, left side if you are left-handed). If it feels contracted, soften it by imagining you are sending your breath there to warm and loosen it. Have the back of your neck long, your face soft, and your hand heavy. Your limbs are heavy and relaxed, your fingers and toes are soft. Your body is heavy and soft. Let your breathing settle to its own comfortable level. It will probably be light and soft.

Imagine that you are standing on a path which leads to the sea.

Notice what the path is like: is it broad and clear? Is it rough or smooth? Is it curved, or straight, or does it have many twists and bends? Are there gates, or obstructions? What is the landscape around you like? What is the weather like? Notice all the details of the scene which came spontaneously into your mind.

Walk along your path towards the sea. Be aware if it is easy or tiring, a short or a long journey. Look at the shore when you arrive at it and again notice the landscape, the weather and the atmosphere.

You are able to swim right down to the depths of the sea. Walk into the sea and swim deep down into the depths. Notice whether it is easy or difficult, notice how you feel, what you see, what the colours, shapes and sensations are.

Now it is time to come out of the sea. If you want to, you can bring something with you. Look around and see what you would like to bring. Take it with you and come out of the sea.

You come out of the sea and onto the shore and find a path which leads to a mountain. What is this path like? Notice what the path is like and notice how you feel. Be aware of the sights and sounds, the weather and the atmosphere. Walk towards the mountain.

You climb to the top of the mountain. Is it easy or difficult? What is the surface of the mountain like to climb on? Notice what you feel like and what you can see and hear.

You arrive at the top of the mountain and sit down for a while. Look around you. Consider how you feel and what you are experiencing. Take your time and observe what is going on for you.

Now it is time to come down from the mountain. If you want to you can bring something with you. Look around and see whether there is anything you would like to take with you. If there is, take it. Come down the mountain again and onto the ground. Perhaps you have something with you from the depths of the sea, and perhaps you have something with you from the top of the mountain.

You are coming along a path which leads you back to your everyday life. How does this feel? Walk back towards your everyday life noticing what you feel, hear and see . . .

Now it is time to bring your awareness back into the room, and to finish your relaxation. Begin to breathe a little more deeply, until you yawn, then yawn a few times. Stretch first your fingers and toes, then your arms and legs, and blink your eyes open to become used to the light. When you are ready, roll over onto your side, push your hands into the floor and sit yourself up.

Take a few moments to collect your thoughts before you return to the activities of your day.

Allow yourself to reflect on the sights, sensations and sounds of your journey and on any objects you 'brought back' with you. Do not search for their 'meaning', but allow any meanings or messages they have for you to evolve in your mind in the days and weeks that follow.

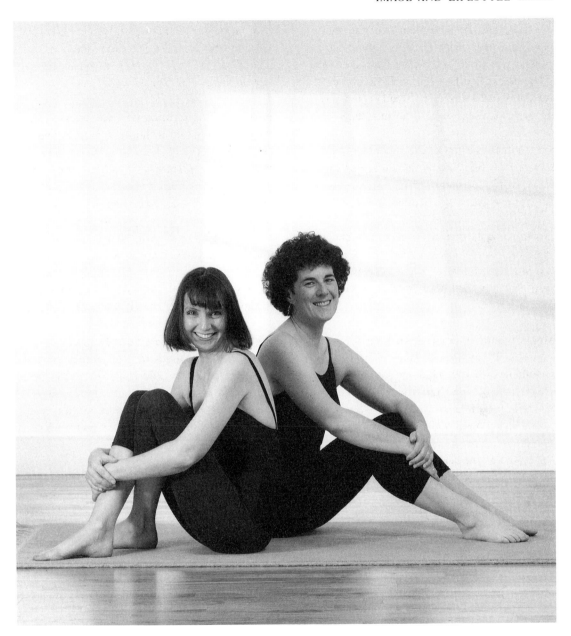

CONCLUSION

In this book we have looked at yoga, at what it might begin to mean and what it might offer to women beginning to consider it as we move towards the twenty-first century.

We have looked at postures which may build and lubricate and liberate the body, and the beginning of work with the breath and with stilling the mind, which may begin to clear the mind of anxiety and bring a growing sense of peace.

We have also looked at awareness and revision of attitudes, and different perspectives on life. There is enough in the practices, the texts and the ideas of yoga to explore for several lifetimes.

It is your own individual choice as to how far you take your own search and research. In your journey you may like finally to bear in mind verse 13 from the *Yoga Sutras*:

The practice of yoga is the commitment to become established in the state of freedom.

FURTHER READING

Effortless Being: The Yoga Sutras of Patanjali, trans. Alistair Shearer, Mandala, 1989

The Upanishads, trans. Shearer and Russell, Mandala, 1989

The Yoga of Light: Hatha-Yoga-Pradipika, trans. and commentary Hans-Ulrich Reiker, Unwin Hyman, 1989

Chakras: Energy Centres of Transformation, Harish Sohari, Destiny Books, 1987

Tao Te Ching (Lao Tzu), trans. Feng and English, Wildwood House, 1986

The Bhagavad Gita, trans. Easwaran, Arkana, 1985

The Dhammapada, trans. Easwaran, Arkana, 1987

Meditations with the Navajo: Navajo Stories of the Earth, Gerald Hausmann, Bear & Co, 1988

Returning to Silence: Zen Practice in Everyday Life, Dainin Katagiri, Shambhala, 1988

Stretch and Relax, Maxine Tobias and Mary Stewart, Dorling Kindersley, 1985

The Book of Yoga, Sivananda Yoga Group, Ebury Press, 1983

Double Yoga, White and Forrest, Penguin, 1981

Pranayama: The Yoga of Breathing, André van Lysbeth, Unwin Hyman, 1979

The Complete Book of Massage, Claire Maxwell-Hudson, Dorling Kindersley, 1988

The Body Has Its Reasons, Thérèse Bertherat, Cedar, 1976

Despair and Personal Power in the Nuclear Age, Joanna Macey, New Society Publishers, USA, 1984

Zen Flesh, Zen Bones: A Collection of Zen and Pre-Zen Writings, ed. Paul Reps, Penguin, 1971

The Hungry Self, Kim Chernin, Virago, 1986

The Art of Starvation: An Adolescent Observed, Sheila Macleod, Virago, 1981

Women and Power – How Far Can We Go?, Nancy Kline, BBC Books, 1992

The Complete Stretching Book, Maxine Tobias and John Patrick Sullivan, Dorling Kindersley, 1992

INDEX

abdominal breathing 29, 50
adolescence 37–8
ageing 58
ahimsa 82
anantasana 54–5
anjaneyasana 49–50, 52
anorexia 77
ardha chandrasana 44

baddha konasana 25
  supta 67
Bhagavadgita 3, 26
bharadvajasana 11, 28
bhujangasana 19
body image 4, 36–7, 51, 56, 75–78

chakras 78–80
chanting 81–2
chatakasana 45
class 2
colours 1, 78–80

dandasana 22
diet 75–78
dragonfly pose 56

Ecclesiastes 51

garudasana 66
gomukhsasana 58
gunas 75–8

halasana 68
hanumanasana 38–9
hatha yoga 1

injuries 2, 16
ishvarapranidhana 86
isolation 59–60

janu sirsasana 54, 62

karnapidasana 68

Lao Tzu 51

mandala 33–4
matsayasana 53
meditation 31–3, 52
menopause 55
menstruation 41–2

natarajasana 73
Niyama 3, 84

Ohm 82

padmasana 41–2
parsvakonasana 12, 61
paschimottanasana 23
Patanjali 3, 91
pelvic floor 48–9
post-natal 51–55
practice 2

pranayama 4, 22, 29
prasarita padottanasana 16
pregnancy 46–51
programme design 6

revitalizing breath 30–31

santosa 35
sarvangasana 28
setu bhandasana 64
stress 65, 66, 69, 70
surya namaskar 69

tadasana 8, 59–60
tapas 85
teachers 2–3, 4
trikonasana 10–11

upavistha konasana 24
urdhva dhanurasana 43
ustrasana 20
uttana padasana 39

vasisthasana 72
virabhadrasan 14, 56, 71
virasana 26
  supta 27
visualization 70, 87
vrksasana 15, 63
vrschikasana 40

yama 3, 82
yantra 33–4
yoga nidra 86

zen 65